· PREVENTION'S ·

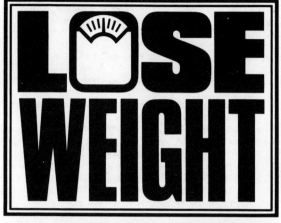

LOSE WEIGHT

GUIDEBOOK

· 1992 ·

Edited by Mark Bricklin
and Anne Remondi Imhoff
of *PREVENTION* Magazine

Rodale Press, Emmaus, Pennsylvania

Chapter 5, "13 Illuminating Tips for Nighttime Snackers," was reprinted by permission of Rawson Associates, an imprint of Macmillan Publishing Company, from "A Baker's Dozen Tips for Night Eaters" in *The I-Don't Eat (But-I-Can't-Lose) Weight Loss Program* by Steven Jonas, M.D., M.P.H., and Virginia Aronson, R.D., M.S. Copyright © 1989 by Steven Jonas and Virginia Aronson.

Chapter 9, "The Perils and Pitfalls of Liquid Fasting Diets," was adapted from "The Grip of the Liquid Diet; A Special Report: Dieters, Craving Balance, Are Battling Fears of Food," by Molly O'Neill, 1 April, 1990. Copyright © 1990 by the New York Times Company. Reprinted by permission.

If you have any questions or comments concerning this book, please write:
Rodale Press
Book Reader Service
33 East Minor Street
Emmaus, PA 18098

ISBN 0-87857-983-4 hardcover

Distributed in the book trade by St. Martin's Press

2 4 6 8 10 9 7 5 3 1   hardcover

Contributors to *Prevention's Lose Weight Guidebook 1992*
Writers: Liz Applegate, Ph.D., Barbara G. Bauer, Ph.D., George L. Blackburn, M.D., Ph.D., Jan Bresnick, Martha Capwell, Virginia DeMoss, Phil Dunphy, Arlene Dym R.D., Stephanie Ebbert, Anne M. Fletcher, M.S., R.D., Denise Foley, Marilee Goldberg, Ph.D., Greg Gutfeld, Chris Hill, Garrett Johnson, Alexis Lieberman, Cemela London, Gale Maleskey, Gloria McVeigh, Jeff Meade, Porter Shimer, Maggie Spilner, Susan Zarrow

Production Editor: Jane Sherman
Designer: Linda Brightbill
Cover Designer: Linda Brightbill
Copy Editor: Sarah Dunn
Executive Editor, *Prevention*
 Magazine: Emrika Padus

Associate Research Chief,
 Prevention Magazine: Pam Boyer
Office Manager: Roberta Mulliner
Office Personnel: Julie Kehs,
 Mary Lou Stephen

Photographers of "After" pictures: Ravell Call (page 185), Tracy Frankel (page 177), Ed Landrock (page 169), Jay Texter (page 165), Stephen Trimble (page 182)

NOTICE

The information and ideas in this book are meant to supplement the care and guidance of your physician, not to replace it. The editor cautions you to see a physician before starting any diet or exercise program. An increasing number of physicians are ready to cooperate with patients who want to improve their diet, health, and lifestyle. If you are under professional care or are taking medication, we suggest discussing any weight-loss plans with your doctor.

Contents

Get ready for a whole new you! Here's your introduction to lifelong weight control and the body
you've always wanted. The good news is that weight
loss and maintenance *are* possible, even if you've
been heavy all your life. Acquaint yourself with this
game plan for victory.

It's the best idea in weight loss to come along in a
long time: Cut fat from your food and melt fat from
your waistline. To do this, you have to know where
the fat is hiding. Here's the lowdown on "low fat"
and your step-by-step formula for eating lean.

Chapter 3: Fight Flab with Fitness:
Get Up, Get Moving!. 65

It's not news that regular exercise is the key to permanent weight loss. What is news: the many different types of exercise to choose from today that make it easier than ever to get started. Now you can choose the kind of activities that are right for you, and learn how to make your exercise burn even more fat and calories.

Chapter 4: The Mind/Body Connection:
How Your Brain Helps Slim Your Body 97

Research has shown that as you confront many of the emotional issues in your life, the pounds begin to peel away. Learning how to overcome the kind of thoughts and feelings that sabotage your diet can shore up your weight loss from the *inside out.*

Chapter 5: The 92 Best Tips of 1992 . . . . **127**

> Here's the best of the bunch—92 quick, easy-to-fol-
> low how-to tips to help you achieve slimming suc-
> cess. Incorporate them into your new healthy life-
> style, and they're sure to help you over the weight-
> loss "humps" and plateaus!

13 Illuminating Tips for Nighttime Snackers • Cooking Right •
Eating Light • Maintain Your Motivation • Mind over Platter •
Beating Binges • How to Harness the Hungries • Fit Bits and
Exercise Tips • Sneak Exercise into Your Life

Chapter 6: Great-Tasting Lean Recipes:
The Perfect Formula for Trimming Down to Size. **145**

> Say good-bye to bland "diet" food and sample our
> collection of this year's best light recipes. They're
> proof that you don't have to deprive yourself of taste
> to lose weight. These dishes offer variety but still
> have plenty in common: They're all healthy and low
> in fat and, most important, they're delicious.

Creole Spinach Salad • Squash Soup • Apricot and Rice Muffins
• Spicy Black Beans • Beans and Rice Combo Plate • Poached
Salmon with Citrus Relish • Pasta with Zucchini and Fresh
Tomatoes • Pizza Dough • Roasted Eggplant and Garlic Pizza
• Delicious Simple Chicken • Sunshine Fruit Shake • Banana-
Strawberry Whip • Berry Crisp

Chapter 7: Profiles of Winners at Losing. **159**

> Following sound principles of sensible eating and
> good health, overweight people can triumph over
> even the toughest, most persistent weight problems.

This chapter features six of this year's most inspirational testimonies, unveiling the winning strategies behind their permanent weight control.

Chapter 8: Answers to Dieters' Most Common Questions

Weight-loss experts answer some of your most troublesome questions. This authoritative, reliable advice is your guide to success.

Confused about the weight-loss gadgets, gizmos, and claims out there? Here's the truth about some of the diet products and services available today. This chapter will dispel a few myths, unveil a few secrets, and help you trim the "fat" from the facts.

Here's your quick-reference guide to the fat and calorie content of hundreds of common foods. And
you're bound to find some surprises. Not all "light"
or "lean" foods are low in fat. And some popular
goodies aren't as fatty as you think!

**Breads • Breakfast Foods • Combination Foods: Dinners and
Entrées • Condiments • Dairy Products • Delicatessen Foods •
Desserts and Sweets • Fast Foods • Fats and Oils • Fish and
Seafood • Frozen Foods • Fruits and Juices • Grain Products •
Meats • Nuts and Seeds • Poultry • Sauces, Gravies, and
Dressings • Snacks • Soups • Vegetables**

Introduction

When Mark Bricklin and I first sat down to discuss the plan for this book, I mentioned my deep personal interest in the subject of weight loss. "I've lost about 50 pounds myself," I admitted, "but it's taken me almost four years to do it."

"Wait a minute," Mark cautioned. "That's kind of like saying, I graduated from college, but it took me four years." Some things are supposed to take time to accomplish. And if they don't, maybe you didn't extract any lasting value from them.

He was right. Permanent weight control requires a type of education. And education takes time. Anyone who has fallen prey to quick weight-loss schemes and diets promising instant results knows this simple truth: In terms of weight loss, the shorter route gets you nowhere fast.

Forget what you may have learned: It's not about will-power or counting calories or self-starvation. Learning how to maintain a slim, healthy body really demands a lifetime commitment, and it also requires that you take a multi-faceted mind and body approach.

So if you think of weight control as an education, there are a number of important lessons to learn. And if you master only one lesson, like reducing your dietary fat, but neglect another, like exercise, it's all too easy to fail.

You should also keep in mind that the weight loss "curriculum" is constantly changing and updating itself. Exciting new research has started to reveal the secrets of reliable weight control. Exercise physiologists, weight-loss psychologists, dietitians, and nutritionists are all homing in on what really works.

How do you personally keep on top of all this ultra-new information? Easy. *Prevention's Lose Weight Guidebook* for 1992 provides you with researchers' latest-breaking discoveries and shows you how to put the information to work in your life.

So roll up your sleeves and open your notebook because you are holding a kind of textbook that will guide you through the inspiring dimensions of your weight-control education.

And finally, remember to be patient with yourself. Read through this book carefully and digest a little of it at a time. It's impossible to learn everything and implement all kinds of changes at once. And it's really self-defeating. Making small but permanent changes is the key to slimming success: buying low-fat milk instead of regular, or walking a few blocks to a friend's house rather than driving. The point is, you're making an educational investment that will last a lifetime, improve your lifetime, and extend your lifetime. And what better investment is there, really, than that?

Anne Imhoff
Coeditor

CHAPTER

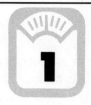

YOUR NEW BODY, YOUR NEW LIFESTYLE

Thin for Life

Everyone has lost weight at one time or another. Some of us have dropped 5 pounds to fit into certain clothes, others have sweated off 50 for a wedding or reunion. But is there anyone out there who's lost weight and kept it off? Not just a few pounds, but real tonnage? And for a long time—more than a year?

You hear it said that 95 percent of all dieters gain their weight back. That can be mighty discouraging to the one out of four Americans considered obese, as well as for yo-yo dieters whose weight bounces up and down. Are the odds really so grim? Is everyone who loses weight doomed to gain it back?

A number of experts interviewed by *Prevention* magazine think not. They say that the statistics on regaining weight are probably distorted by the toughest obesity cases—people who've failed at weight loss time and time again and who have the most to lose. They're the very people who are likely to be attracted to research centers that publish studies whose statistics get quoted.

Also, several experts suspect that many people who do lose weight and keep it off on their own never "make it" into published statistics because they never sign up at research programs.

And this suspicion that there are more weight-loss success stories out there than people think is backed up by some compelling research. Several years ago, renowned obesity researcher Stanley Schachter, Ph.D., at Columbia University, had a hunch that "obesity's reputation for intractability" was grossly exaggerated. He also suspected that many people lose weight—and keep it off—on their own. To confirm his hypotheses, he quizzed 161 people—both in his psychology department and at a summer resort—about their efforts at weight loss.

Dr. Schachter's conclusion: The rate of self-cure of obesity (which he defined as being 15 percent or more overweight) was "considerably higher than any yet reported in the literature." He found that of the 46 people who had a history of obesity, 25 would be considered successfully cured—that is, they were no longer fat and had stayed that way for some time. On average, the reducers had lost 34.7 pounds and had maintained their losses for about 11 years.

Dr. Schachter's survey was informal, and his subjects may not have represented the general population. But his findings were soon affirmed by a study published by two other researchers in the *Journal of Addictive Behaviors*. Robert Colvin, Ph.D., and Susan Olson, Ph.D., recruited and interviewed people who had lost 20 percent or more of their body weight. "Success" was defined as having kept the weight off—to within 5 pounds of their lowest weight—for at least two years.

Through radio, newspaper, and television publicity, the researchers were able to track down 41 women who had lost and kept off an average of about 53 pounds for six years. They also interviewed 13 men who had maintained an average loss of 76 pounds for about the same period of time. And only 21 of these 54 "big losers" had reduced with the help of weight-loss programs or medical supervision.

Apparently there's even hope of permanent weight loss for people who've been heavy most of their lives. Several of the "walking success stories" who were interviewed were either overweight when they were young or came from overweight families. Kerry Kaplan says, "Every recipe my mother made started with a stick of butter. My father, sisters, and brothers are horribly obese." But he has kept off 50 pounds for the past five years. Then about a year ago he took off the other 50 he needed to lose. Now his weight is at 176, down 106 pounds from his all-time high.

Kerry freely admits that for him weight maintenance is a lot of work, but he has beaten the odds stacked against him by his family history. "The effort I have to put in," he says, "is only one one-hundredth the psychic pain of being 100 pounds overweight."

How-to Strategies for Lifelong Weight Control

So just what are Kerry and others doing that has helped them drop—and never regain—unwanted pounds?

That's exactly what this book is all about. We've collected solid evidence from the latest breakthoughs in the science of weight loss. We've interviewed the experts and heard testimony from winners in the war against fat. Here's an overview of the game plan for victory.

Squeeze the Fat out of Your Diet

Successful weight maintenance doesn't necessarily mean eating like a bird and feeling deprived. It can mean eating your fill—of low-fat cuisine. Many long-term maintainers have learned how to ensure that their low-fat eating is high in satisfaction and low on boredom. They create new low-fat dishes with lean meats, fish, chicken, vegetables, whole grains, and fruit. They experiment with herbs and spices. They try new low-fat recipes (like those featured in chapter 6). Among the successful maintainers in a study by psychologist Judith Rodin, Ph.D., head of the Psychology Department at Yale University, low-fat eating and cooking had become more than a dietary requirement—it was fun.

But making the change to low-fat eating takes a little practice. You'll need to know exactly what to buy, and you will have to start taking a better look at the labels of your favorite foods. Check out chapter 2, which features a consumer's guide to low-fat shopping that will get you off to a good start.

Go for moderation, not denial. Most of the successful people who were interviewed by *Prevention,* as well as the maintainers in a study conducted by registered dietitian Susan Kayman, Dr.P.H., and *Prevention* adviser Judith Stern, Sc.D., and a colleague, did not forbid themselves favorite foods. They simply ate these in moderation. In contrast, relapsers tended to deny themselves enjoyable foods while dieting. Some weight-control experts believe that banning specific foods from your eating is actually self-defeating.

Get Moving

Without hesitation, every expert interviewed said that regular exercise distinguishes successful maintainers from relapsers. And a study in the *American Journal of Clinical Nutrition* heartily supports this view. In the research, Dr. Kayman and Dr. Stern compared 30 women who had maintained weight loss to 44 relapsers. And guess what: 90 percent of the maintainers said they exercised regularly (at least three times a week for half an hour or more), while only 34 percent of regainers did so.

But for exercise to be effective in maintaining weight loss, do you really have to knock yourself out? No, say the experts. According to *Prevention* adviser Kelly Brownell, Ph.D., co-director of the University of Pennsylvania Obesity Research Clinic, and Dr. Rodin, what's most important is exercising on a regular basis. It's got to become part of your routine, just like brushing your teeth.

Adjust Your Attitude

It's important to "look out for number one." Dr. Colvin and Dr. Olson found that, in general, their successful maintainers learned to do a better job of meeting their own needs. They attended to their home and family but also made time for themselves, for personal pampering, for career and other pursuits.

And while relapsers said they avoided confronting crises and instead used food to make themselves feel better when upset, the eight maintainers in Dr. Kayman's study were more likely to deal with problems directly and to use problem-solving skills in coping with day-to-day crises. "Say you get up to go to work one morning and your kid falls and starts bleeding," says Dr. Stern. "Then your babysitter cancels. Next the car breaks down. Our successful maintainers were more likely to deal with such problems in order of priority rather than panic."

"I know I overeat when I'm stressed," says Tom Frank, who has lost 55 pounds and kept it off for 15 years. "But when I accept the problem and do something about it, the overeating disappears."

It's also important to check your weight occasionally and have a plan of action if it's unacceptable. That doesn't mean you have to weigh yourself compulsively. Some people go by the fit of their clothes. Others have a weight goal or range that they view as acceptable. If your weight goes above your limits, activate your strategy to get the pounds off again. You may go back to a group program like Weight Watchers. Or you might reread the book that helped you lose weight in the first place. Some people double their exercise.

Go slow and steady. Dr. Rodin and Michaela Kiernan conducted one of the handful of studies ever done on successful maintenance of weight loss. What struck these researchers about the regainers in their study was that they were "very much on or off."

"For a while they ate well and exercised, going all out, then they went back to their old ways," says Dr. Rodin. But the maintainers didn't feel that they had to throw themselves into their weight-control regimen with a vengeance. They preferred a more realistic effort—and were consistent about it. They might have exercised only three times a week, but they did it consistently.

To adopt this strategy, you'll have to stop thinking of your improved eating habits as a "diet." Long-term weight loss means getting rid of the "diet mentality," the notion that you're simply jumping into yet another artificial—and probably temporary—regimen. The experts agree: You have to view weight control as a permanent, lifelong process.

Nearly everyone *Prevention* interviewed had spent years on the diet merry-go-round. Kerry Kaplan exclaims, "You name the diet, I've been on it." But when he and others like him finally accepted their weight-control strategies as a way of life (not a short-term experiment), they succeeded. Their weight loss was usually slow and gradual, taking years rather than weeks or months to reach their weight goals. It was a lasting solution, not a quick fix.

The research conducted by Dr. Kayman and her co-investigators at Kaiser Permanente Medical Center in Fremont, California, seems to support the wisdom of this "in for the long haul" attitude. They found that maintainers, unlike regainers, were aware that they needed to continue indefinitely to be conscious of the amount and type of food they consumed, as well as their level of activity, if they wanted to keep their weight down.

Another important factor is support. Dr. Brownell likens the needs of some (but not all) "recovered" obese people to recovered alcoholics. "They may well need some sort of lifelong group support to keep the weight off forever," he says. Certain people do best in an organized weight-loss group. Others work well with a buddy system—that is, working with a partner who's also trying to keep the weight off.

Before You Begin

Two of every three men are happy with their body weight, according to a poll, compared to just one of every two women. Where do you fit in that group? It's important to be sure you *want* to lose weight before embarking on a weight-loss plan.

"Everybody's got to determine his own readiness," says Nancy Cohen, Ph.D., a registered dietitian and assistant professor of nutrition at the University of Massachusetts. She adds that it's how you perceive your weight-loss plan that often makes all the difference: The trick is to change your eating and exercise habits—habits that you have to slowly incorporate into your lifestyle.

Set Your "Diet Alarm Clock" for 12 Weeks
By George L. Blackburn, M.D., Ph.D.

associate professor of surgery at Harvard Medical School and chief of the Nutrition/Metabolism Laboratory with the Cancer Research Institute at New England Deaconess Hospital, Boston.

The latest scoop on weight loss: A little loss goes a long way, even if you have a lot to lose. How can that be? There are two reasons. First, weight loss is easier and far more likely to be permanent when it starts with one small step. You'll lose more in the long run if you start by losing just a little, then give yourself a good, long rest. And second, those first few pounds you lose are the ones that have the biggest health payoff.

So if you're about to give weight loss a try, jot down this magic number: 12. In our research at New England Deaconess Hospital, we've made an important discovery: The body wants to lose weight for only about 12 weeks. Then it doesn't want to budge for quite a while, and if you force it, you're more likely to burn out, go off the diet, and start overeating again.

A lot of people diet for six months at a time or even a year. But we recommend that people stop dieting after 12 weeks and "rest" for several months, even if they have more weight to lose. It gives their body time to adjust to the new "set point" (the weight your metabolism is geared to hold) before attempting another descent.

This is critical, because what makes weight loss so difficult is that your body tries to defend its old set point. Careening from a high set point down to an "ideal body weight" is more difficult than descending step by step, giving the body a chance to reset gradually.

By dropping about 1 to 2 pounds a week—the safest rate of weight loss—you could easily take off 15 pounds in those 12 weeks. But suppose you need to lose 50 to reach the standard for your height and build (as shown on weight tables on page 13)? Don't you have to keep going to reap the health benefits of weight loss? The good news here is that, according to our research, when you lose those first 15 pounds, you immediately glean about 75 percent of the health benefits of losing the full 50.

Reaping the Emotional Rewards

We've found that dropping just 30 percent of your excess weight can bring a significant decrease in the health risks associated with obesity and can bring a sizable boost in your quality of life to boot. We studied thousands of dieters. As they lost weight, we measured their blood pressure, their serum cholesterol, and their blood sugar levels, as well as other elements like sleep, stamina, and clothing size. The medical tests gave us an idea of their risk for cardiovascular disease, hypertension, diabetes, gastrointestinal disorders, and other obesity-related problems. The other measurements told us about their quality of life. We found that by the time people have lost about 30 percent of their excess weight (which is usually about 5 to 15 percent of their total body weight), they have achieved 70 to 80 percent of the health and quality-of-life benefits! People feel much better, and their disease risk is significantly reduced through moderate weight loss.

Other good reasons to start small with weight loss: It's easy to achieve a 10- to 15-pound weight loss by eating just a little less and exercising just a little more.

And even this small weight reduction changes your metabolism. It can lower blood pressure, elevated blood fats, and the body's demand for insulin.

Being overweight stresses your body. You're eating too much and, usually, not moving enough. Your body struggles to metabolize the excess food and has to work harder to do just about anything because you're unfit and sedentary. When you lose just a few pounds by eating a little less and moving about a little more, the balance between eating and activity shifts to a more beneficial level. Your body has less food to metabolize and less weight to lug around. A burden is lifted immediately. That's why people often feel exhilarated after being on this kind of weight-loss program for just a short time.

Losing just 10 to 15 pounds can improve your ability to do pleasurable leisure activities that help you burn even more calories. You're more interested in taking walks, going to museums, and traveling.

Unfortunately, people who need to lose almost always focus on the total amount they should drop to reach a svelte ideal. That number can often be daunting. They take off a few pounds, get discouraged, and start overeating again. Or worse, they're so impatient to lose all the extra weight that they go on a crash diet. It comes off quickly, all right—but before long, it's back.

As you can see, people who are 30 to 50 pounds overweight can benefit enormously by devoting three months to losing just 10 to 15 pounds. People who are less than 30 pounds overweight can benefit by losing even less.

To achieve and sustain a 10- to 15-pound weight loss, you need to cut only 100 to 150 calories a day—not too difficult. Vigorous activity, like brisk walking, chores, or gardening, burns about 5 calories a minute. So if you wanted to burn all the calories through exercise, you'd have to do about 20 to 30 extra minutes of activity a day (above your current level).

Once you've lost the 10 or 15 pounds, stay at that set-point level for six months to a year. Then you can think about whether you need another 12-week session to lose another 10 to 15 pounds.

Keep your weight-loss goals small, and slowly but surely you'll feel better, look better, and permanently shed the pounds that weigh you down.

Your Ideal Weight: Closer Than You Think

So, what's your goal, your target "ideal" weight?

When asked, most people over 40 would probably choose a weight from their twenties or thirties, when they really looked and felt good. But experts tell us that's history; what counts more than numbers on a scale is the percentage and distribution of your body fat.

"Ideal" in these terms means 20 to 30 percent fat for women in their forties and 15 to 25 percent for men—something that can only be ascertained with specialized tests and trained personnel available at some health clubs.

Also to be considered is where the fat is located. Research shows that fat gained in the upper body—arms, shoulders, neck, and waist especially—appears to entail more health risks than fat that accumulates in the areas of the hips, buttocks, and thighs. Better to be a pear, in other words, than a pumpkin.

"We also need to distinguish between cosmetic considerations and what's appropriate for reasons of comfort and health," says Reubin Andres, M.D., clinical director of the National Institute on Aging. "Some of us were born greyhounds and others of us were born bulldogs. It may not be advisable to try too hard to change our nature."

George L. Blackburn, M.D., Ph.D., associate professor of surgery at Harvard Medical School and chief of the Nutrition/Metabolism Laboratory with the Cancer Research Institute at New England Deaconess Hospital, Boston, agrees. "We shouldn't be led by our nostalgic yearnings to weigh what we did in high school, or by desire to look like ultraskinny fashion models."

A healthy weight is, quite simply, one you can maintain by eating a nutritious low-fat diet and exercising daily—the kind of program outlined in this book. Now, that's certainly something to think about, especially if your personal Battle of the Bulge so far has been a losing struggle.

A More Tolerant Table

If you're the kind of person who needs a particular ideal weight, in numbers, to focus your weight-loss efforts, you'll be pleased to learn that authorities have developed a much more tolerant weight table. New government dietary guidelines have much broader limits than previous ones, and they also consider age, not just height, in determining a healthy weight (after age 35, they cut you a 10- to 15-pound break).

The higher weights in the ranges generally apply to men, who tend to have more muscle and bone; the lower weights more often apply to women, who have less muscle and bone. The new ranges are shown in the table on the opposite page.

That M & M Is 100 Yards Long

It takes one football field of walking to burn off one little M & M candy, according to physiologist Robert

SUGGESTED WEIGHTS FOR ADULTS   ◆

HEIGHT	WEIGHT IN POUNDS	
	19–34 YEARS	35 YEARS AND OVER
5'0"	97–128	108–138
5'1"	101–132	111–143
5'2"	104–137	115–148
5'3"	107–141	119–152
5'4"	111–146	122–157
5'5"	114–150	126–162
5'6"	118–155	130–167
5'7"	121–160	134–172
5'8"	125–164	138–178
5'9"	129–169	142–183
5'10"	132–174	146–188
5'11"	136–179	151–194
6'0"	140–184	155–199
6'1"	144–189	159–205
6'2"	148–195	164–210
6'3"	152–200	168–216
6'4"	156–205	173–222
6'5"	160–211	177–228
6'6"	164–216	182–234

NOTE: Height measured without shoes; weight measured without clothes.

Neeves, Ph.D., coauthor of *The Walking Off Weight Workbook.*

To give yourself a sense of how a large amount of walking burns a tiny amount of fat, Dr. Neeves recommends you buy a small bag of plain M & M's and take it to a football field. Eat one M & M and walk the entire length of the football field—end zones included. When you reach the other end, ask yourself, "If I eat this M & M, would I be willing to walk the length of this field again?"

If the answer is no, throw away your M & M's and go home. If the answer is yes, eat the M & M and walk one more football field. Then, at the other end, ask yourself again, "Am I willing to walk another football field for another M & M?"

Repeat the procedure until you're out of candy, whether it's because you threw it out or because you ate it all. If you ate the whole bagful, you walked 55 lengths of the football field, which is about 3.3 miles.

The point isn't to count every calorie you eat against every calorie you burn. "Not all the food we eat needs to be walked off," writes Dr. Neeves. "In the normal course of daily living your resting metabolism operates at 800 to 1,200 calories per day just to maintain normal body functions."

This exercise merely shows how much energy is stored in even small amounts of fat. So you can imagine how much energy is in large chunks of fat. A Big Mac, fries, and a shake are equivalent to 240 football fields. If you don't walk the 5 hours it takes to go that distance, guess what happens to that energy? That's right, it gets stuffed into your fat cells.

It's just one more example to underscore the importance of eating low-fat foods and getting regular exercise. And that's what your new lifestyle is all about!

Food Cravings Linked to a Pleasure Chemical

Chemically speaking, food cravings may be kissing cousins to that far more serious craving, an addiction to heroin. In one study, Adam Drewnowski, Ph.D., director of human nutrition at the University of Michigan, injected nine women with naloxone, a "pleasure-killer" drug that is used to prevent heroin from being absorbed by the brain when people take overdoses. The drug had the same impact on cravings for food as it had on cravings for heroin: It stopped cravings for fats and sweets. When offered a selection of foods to eat, including chocolate and cookies, the naloxone-injected women ate *59 percent fewer dietary fat calories* than women who did not receive the naloxone.

What's going on? Well, when we eat sweets or fats, the body produces pleasure chemicals called opioids. But the naloxone blocks the ability of these opioids to deliver their message of pleasure to the brain. And no pleasure equals no craving.

As further proof, Dr. Drewnowski turned the experiment around. He injected another group of women with *extra* pleasure chemicals in the form of a drug called butorphanol. These women reported more pleasure from the taste of fats and sweets.

"This study suggests that our physiological mechanism for food cravings may be the same as that for drug addictions," says Dr. Drewnowski.

However, don't think a cure for cravings is around the corner. "One major newspaper ran an article on this study, saying we 'found a way to break the vicious cycle of addiction to M & M candies.' It's not true. This study is preliminary; naloxone is not available to the public to block food cravings and is too short-lasting to make a difference anyway. But this research may *lead* to solutions, once we better understand the mechanisms of cravings."

Dr. Drewnowski is now studying people who say they have cravings for sweets and fats to see if they have an exaggerated response to opioids.

Just Add Water and Reduce Water Retention

A major reason for overeating is that we think our body is crying out for food when it is actually crying out for water. So next time you feel like eating, drink water. Not only could it water down your cravings, it can also help you look slimmer!

When water intake is too meager (usually under eight cups a day), the body will secrete the hormone aldosterone, which causes the body to hold on to every molecule of water and sodium it can, according to *Fat, Water Retention and You,* by the late Peter Lindner, M.D.

It makes biological sense because when there's a drought, you need every drop of water you can get. Water retention is especially pronounced if protein intake is too low (often the case in fad diets) and/or there is an estrogen imbalance, as there is right before menstruation.

So a person with normal kidney and heart function actually needs to drink more water to get rid of excess fluid. This decreases the production of aldosterone and stimulates excretion of water.

By drinking more water each day to meet your optimal water needs, you will reach the "breakthrough point." You will definitely know you have reached it by sudden loss of signs of fluid retention, a sudden loss of weight of several pounds, and a normal thirst.

Although much individual variation exists, basic water intake needs are 10 to 12 8-ounce glasses of water per day. If you are overweight, then you need to drink one extra glass for every 25 pounds above your ideal body weight.

A Point for Purists

If you're planning to stock up on your favorite variety of bottled water, you may want to reconsider. Plain tap water is usually better than more expensive bottled waters, report researchers at Northeastern University. The reason? Most bottled water is not refrigerated (particularly during the shipping process), and when it is stored at room temperature for 30 days, bacteria can increase anywhere from 100-fold to 10,000-fold.

Although tap water isn't refrigerated either, these bacteria are usually killed when chlorine or ozone is added to local drinking supplies. Advice: If you drink bottled water, keep it refrigerated for several days before consumption.

Added Payoffs for Shedding the Pounds

Being attractive pays off—literally. A study by the University of Pittsburgh finds that "good-looking" job applicants in marketing, sales, and data processing typically receive a starting salary of $2,200 more than a candidate who is equally qualified but not as attractive. Overweight men can also expect salaries $2,000 lower than slimmer people with the same credentials, although weight had no effect on women's pay.

Nathan Pritikin: A Pioneer of the Weight-Control Lifestyle

Founded more than a decade ago, the Pritikin Longevity Centers have helped thousands lose weight and reduce their risk of heart disease. And not with drugs or bypass surgery—with lifestyle changes.

Pritikin's therapeutic lifestyle regimen was quite revolutionary at the time: a very-low-fat diet (less than 10 percent of calories from fat), regular aerobic exercise, and stress management. But since then, its stunning results have been published in respectable cardiology journals. No small feat, considering its humble beginnings.

Nathan Pritikin, the Centers' founder, wasn't a cardiologist; indeed, he had no medical training whatsoever. He was a self-educated engineer who in 1957 was diagnosed with arterial blockage so severe his doctor advised him to make sure his life insurance was paid up. Unfortunately, in the fat-laden 1950s, doctors knew little about the connection between diet and heart health.

But during World War II, Pritikin happened to be privy to military medical research that suggested a link.

At that time, stress was generally considered the major cause of heart disease. But a military-funded study disclosed that, despite the stress experienced by people in war-torn Europe, the incidence of heart attacks actually declined.

Pritikin had a hunch that diet was the key factor. World War II had created famine conditions: Meat, butter and cream were in short supply; baked goods were but sweet memories. People had no choice but to eat an extremely low-fat diet.

And so, against his doctor's "better judgment," Pritikin declared war on heart disease. He put himself on a very-low-fat, high-fiber diet and started exercising. In short order, he cut his serum cholesterol from nearly 300 to 120 and, with it, his risk of a heart attack.

With his personal success as a model, Pritikin proceeded to preach what he practiced, in books and later at the Longevity Centers.

Today, research conducted by Dean Ornish, M.D., director of the Preventive Medicine Research Institute in Sausalito, and others supports the heart-healthy benefits of a program including low-fat diet and exercise.

The Pritikin Eating Plan

The Pritikin people don't call their program a "diet" anymore, not officially, anyway. They prefer the term "Lifetime Eating Plan" (LEP), because it suggests the kind of gradual, gentle, but lasting improvements they feel will work best.

The LEP suggests the following guidelines for daily food intake:

• Two servings of nonfat yogurt or skim milk
• Six to eight servings of vegetables
• Three to four whole fruits

• Four to five servings of unrefined complex carbohydrates like whole-grain bread, pasta, rice, beans, peas, or potatoes
• One 3½-ounce serving of lean meat or fish

The Pritikin Lifetime Eating Plan calls for a decrease in total fat intake to 10 percent or less of total calories (compared to the 35 to 45 percent of the typical Western diet), no more than 100 milligrams of cholesterol and 1,600 milligrams of sodium per day, and at least 40 grams of fiber every day.

The goal of this plan is to achieve a total cholesterol of 100 points plus your age, with 160 being the maximum. "Almost nobody with a long-term cholesterol level below 160 develops heart disease," says Monroe Rosenthal, M.D., medical director of the Santa Monica Pritikin Center.

As a quick guide, every Pritikin participant receives a pamphlet that divides foods into three categories: Go, Caution, and Stop.

• *Go* foods are fully recommended and include fresh fruits, vegetables, whole grains, nonfat dairy products, legumes, chestnuts, fish, and lean fowl or lean red meat—all in suggested amounts.
• *Caution* foods, in small amounts, pose little danger, and include decaffeinated coffee and tea, sweeteners such as honey and molasses, low-sodium soy sauce and miso, low-fat dairy products, monounsaturated and polyunsaturated oils, unsalted nuts, avocados, and olives.
• *Stop* foods will significantly raise the risk of heart disease. These include butter, tropical oils, mayonnaise, foods with animal fats, fatty meats, whole dairy products, salt, coconuts, macadamia nuts, egg yolks, and fried foods.

Says Dr. Rosenthal, "The goal is not to divide your life into 'staying on the program' and 'cheating,' but to make choices. You're never 'off' the program, you just make choices that are poor, better, or best."

How about losing weight? Does the Lifetime Eating Plan melt the pounds away?

"This is a slow, consistent weight-loss program," says Dr. Rosenthal. "You will see more rapid weight loss with other programs, up to twice as fast. But on those programs your appetite increases and you usually regain the weight rapidly.

"We don't want you to focus on losing as much weight as quickly as you can. The goal here is to look, feel, and be healthy. And all the research we've seen and performed suggests that a diet high in unrefined complex carbohydrates, low in fat, high in fiber, and low in cholesterol, plus exercise (which we define as a daily walking program) will bring about the best improvements—in both heart health and weight loss."

The plan also includes stress management, which Dr. Rosenthal sums up as "Don't get too hungry, angry, lonely, or tired. These are the times you eat. Plan ahead."

Documented Proof

Pritikin is a pricey program: over $5,000 for 13 days; over $8,000 for 26 days (less than 20 percent is eligible for coverage by medical insurance). But those who can afford it say it's worth it. The Pritikin Research Foundation has published more than 20 studies that collectively demonstrate that the Pritikin program may, in two to four weeks:

• Lower cholesterol and triglycerides by 25 percent.
• Reduce high blood pressure and the need for hypertension medications. In a study of over 200 Pritikin participants, 83 percent who entered the program while taking high blood pressure medication were able to normalize their blood pressure without drugs.

• Decrease angina pain and the need for angina medication. In one study, angina patients who could walk only about ½ mile a day were walking an average of 5½ miles each day when they left the four-week program. In another study, 62 percent were able to leave their cardiac medication behind when they completed the program.

• Help avoid bypass surgery. Eighty percent of 64 patients who were slated for bypass, but chose to attend the Pritikin program instead, had not had the operation five years later.

• Help weight loss. Overweight people have lost an average of 13 pounds during the 26-day program.

• Reduce dependence on insulin. In one study, over 50 percent of Type-II diabetics on insulin left the program free of the drug, and over 90 percent on oral drugs left drug-free.

Going the Distance: Exercise Strategies to Keep You on Track

Since regular exercise is one of the cornerstones of the Pritikin program, the staff has assembled a few pointers to help you maintain your personal routine.

Set realistic goals. If it's clear why you're exercising, and if you can see the results, you're more likely to stick with it. Begin with short-term goals, such as losing a few pounds or feeling better. These can be used as a bridge to goals that take longer to achieve, such as changes in body composition or improvements in blood chemistry.

Solicit the support of family and friends. Let those who are close to you know how important your exercise program is to you—and that you'd appreciate their cooperation and support in helping you achieve your goals.

Purchase home exercise equipment. Make no excuses: Exercising at home is convenient. You can do it at any time and in any weather if you have a treadmill, stationary bike, or mini-trampoline.

Join a fitness club. Fitness clubs, with their variety of exercise options, are a great way to keep your exercise routine from getting boring.

Record your progress. Keep a log of your daily workouts. Include such details as speed and duration of the workout, heart rate, and perceived level of exertion and discomfort. You'll gain pride and encouragement from seeing your progress on paper. Also, keeping track of how many pounds and inches you've lost can help motivate you to stay with your program.

Foster a positive mental attitude. If you enjoy your exercise, you'll look forward to it and maintain it. So emphasize the positive aspects: how much better you feel, how much weight you've lost, how much healthier you are. And don't forget to enjoy the scenery and the companionship of your exercise partners, too.

Keep the benefits of exercise in mind. Remind yourself of all the good you're doing by exercising: strengthening your heart, normalizing your blood pressure, decreasing body fat and increasing lean body mass, increasing overall strength, increasing HDL cholesterol, and elevating your mood.

Smart Cooking for a Healthy Heart

Susan Masseron, who teaches two cooking classes a day at the Pritikin Center in Santa Monica, acknowledges that some convenience foods are just fine. "We want you to be able to stay on the diet easily...so everything doesn't have to be pulled up by the roots or still have feathers on it," she says. Still, this is a new way of cooking. The following are some of the tips collected during those classes, while waiting to sample the delicious dishes that Masserson created. No one ever left early.

Learn to make yogurt "cream cheese." For a fat-free substitute for cream cheese and sour cream, this is unbeatable. Simply line a strainer with three layers of cheesecloth and fill with a quart of nonfat yogurt. Set it in a bowl in the refrigerator to drain overnight. In the morning you'll have creamy, nonfat cheese, which you can mix with nonfat milk, raisins, dates, chives, or dill.

Use chicken stock instead of oil for sautéing. Masserson recommends defatting chicken stock by first leaving it in the refrigerator overnight, then skimming off the fat in the morning, after it has congealed. The stock can then be strained through cheesecloth and frozen in an ice-cube tray, which provides convenient cubes for sautéing.

Rinse canned food to remove salt. You can get rid of as much as half of the salt in canned beans and vegetables by rinsing them before using.

Use herbs and spices to replace salt and oil. Cooking without salt and oil can leave your taste buds wondering where the flavor went—at least until they adjust back to the natural flavors of foods. Fresh herbs, however, can open up a tasty new world. Good markets often carry fresh herbs such as basil, dill, parsley, mint, garlic, chives, and cilantro.

Freeze bite-size fruit chunks for snacks. Seedless grapes are the easiest, but peaches, pears, melons, and bananas provide a satisfying snack when frozen.

How to "Insure" Your Weight Loss

"Five years ago, health insurance companies wouldn't reimburse any treatment related to obesity," says Janet McBarron, M.D., who chairs the American Society of Bariatric Physicians (ASBP) Insurance Relations Committee. "But that's changing as it is increasingly clear that obesity is related to heart disease and diabetes—[former] Surgeon General Koop announced that 70 percent of people die prematurely because of what they eat. So now, [some] companies pay up to 100 percent of the costs for weight-loss programs."

It's still not easy to get an insurance company to pay for weight loss. But it can be possible if you satisfy the following criteria.

You're 100 pounds or more overweight. This much excess poundage is often considered a medical problem that requires treatment.

You're treating an associated condition. "Obesity itself is not considered an illness or a disease, so we [Blue Cross/Blue Shield] don't pay for treatment of obesity," says William Rial, M.D., director of provider services (health benefits division) of the National Association of Blue Cross/Blue Shield in Chicago. "However, if weight reduction is part of a treatment for hypertension, diabetes mellitus, traumatic arthritis of weight-bearing joints, pulmonary insufficiency, or Pickwickian syndrome [a genetic form of obesity], we can pay for covered benefits."

"You may think weight is your only problem, but weight can be related to so many things that are covered in insurance," adds Dr. McBarron. "That's why it's a good idea to get a checkup from a bariatric physician. You may have an associated problem such as high cholesterol, high blood pressure, or a thyroid condition and not know it. And if you're feeling depressed because of your weight, insurance may pay for therapy, because depression is a medical disease."

You go to a doctor or a hospital-based program. Most insurance companies don't pay for commercial programs, such as Weight Watchers or Nutri/System. Since they pay only for medical conditions, they want a medical doctor supervising the process. "You stand a better chance of being reimbursed if you choose a board-certified doctor from the ASBP," says Dr. McBarron. "Insurance companies don't want to pay for any doctor who just passes out amphetamines or a diet sheet. A doctor from the ASBP is required to practice a more thorough treatment plan."

Don't assume that you're out of luck on the insurance front, though; check on your coverage, or change coverage if necessary.

Ask your employer if weight loss is covered. Some companies include weight loss on their insurance plan, just as they may opt to pay such benefits as maternity coverage or eye care.

Ask the insurance underwriter up front. "And be careful how you word your inquiry," says Dr. McBarron. "If you ask them if they'll pay for weight loss, nine out of ten will say no. Instead, describe the associated conditions, explain you're going to see a doctor, and ask how much is covered. And make sure you get the name of the underwriter in case you run into any problems later."

Sign up for an HMO. Health Maintenance Organizations, or HMOs, make contracts with specific weight-loss groups, such as Weight Watchers or Diet Workshop. You don't have a wide choice of which one to attend, but they pay 100 percent of the costs.

Beware the Age of the Bulge

Warning: The years between ages 25 and 34 may be hazardous to your belt. That's the time you're most likely to put on the extra pounds, according to a study by the Department of Health and Human Services.

In the ten-year study, researchers monitored the weights of 10,000 men and women aged 25 to 74. They found not only that weight gain was highest for both men and women between 25 and 34, but also that women were twice as likely as men to experience major weight gain (30 pounds or more). Women younger than 45 who were overweight to begin with had an even greater chance of major weight gain during the ten years of the study. Interestingly, after men and women reached the age of 55, their weight began to drop slightly.

"There are a lot of middle-aged people with weight problems, but these problems develop early on," says researcher David F. Williamson, Ph.D., of the Centers for Disease Control in Atlanta (division of nutrition). "A weight gain of 30 pounds or more over a short period of time is dangerous. But so is simply being overweight—especially for women. It's well proven that excess weight increases your risk for high blood pressure, heart disease, and diabetes." (To figure your ideal weight, see page 13.)

Dr. Williamson suggests you adopt healthy habits early to head off potential weight gain later in life. "Weight control shouldn't start when you're 55. People should consider exercise like walking, which, if done regularly, will help prevent the accumulation of excess fat." He also stresses the importance of a diet rich in fruits and vegetables and low in fat—the kind of food highlighted in our field guide to low-fat shopping on page 31. More research is under way.

Watch for Early Warning Signs: You're About to Gain

Maintaining your weight has to become a habit. Until exercise and eating a low-fat, high-fiber diet are natural parts of your lifestyle, maintenance is work.

"From our thousands of patients, we have gleaned a short list of flashing yellow lights, warning signals of impending abandonment of all best-laid plans to lose weight," says Maria Simonson, Ph.D., Sc.D., director of the Health, Weight, and Stress Program at Johns Hopkins Medical Institutions in Baltimore, and author of *The Complete University Medical Diet.*

"When you spot any of these signs, watch out. Start using positive thinking, stress reduction, or motivation techniques that have helped you. Don't let inertia and an urge to let nature take its course ('I told you, I have no willpower') block your intentions to improve your body."

Here are the signs that you need to take action.

• You compare yourself to other people who are losing more weight on the same calories or people who don't have to watch their calories. You feel envious or angry and terribly deprived.

• You are spending an unusual amount of time watching television.

• You have cravings for specific foods.

• You start skipping breakfast (or lunch) again.

• Strolling past a bakery or a delicatessen, you decide to go in and buy some treats for the family. You're not going to eat any, of course.

• You start blaming your husband, your mother-in-law, your cat, your boss, or your children for annoying and upsetting you so much that you are getting urges to eat foods you know you shouldn't.

• You notice you are watching other people eat.

• You're discouraged because you hardly lost any weight this week despite adherence to your diet plan.

• People are beginning to notice your weight loss and to say, "You are looking marvelous. You're losing weight, aren't you?" This is the moment when many people allow their fear of thinness to overwhelm their desire to become what they have always wanted to be—thin.

• You start to cheat a little here and there, thinking, "What does it matter, this tiny piece of cake?" Or you increase your portions.

CHAPTER

LIVING THE
LOW-FAT LIFE

Fighting Fat Beats Counting Calories

Are you carefully counting your calories but not *maintaining* your weight loss? Consider changing your approach. Encouraging new research suggests that fat reduction can help keep weight off with fewer fluctuations than a traditional calorie-counting diet. Fifty-one overweight men and women were randomly assigned to low-fat or low-calorie test diets for four to five months. The low-fat group cut back fat intake to about 1 ounce per day, with no other calorie restrictions. The low-calorie group was on a strict diet (1,200 calories per day for women; 1,500 for men), cutting both fat and carbohydrate intake.

Individuals in the low-calorie group lost more weight (an average of 21.6 pounds versus 12.3 pounds) during the study than those who restricted only fat. But they also gained more weight back after the study ended. At a 9- to 12-month follow-up, the low-fat group had gained back much less weight, on average, than the low-calorie group (the low-fat group had regained an average of 3.3 pounds; the low-calorie group regained an average of 13 pounds). The low-fat group is the one that actually came out ahead. They didn't lose as much at first but, unlike the calorie-restricted group, they managed to keep most of it off—the *real* goal of a successful weight-loss plan.

Now more than ever before, diet experts are convinced that reducing dietary fat plays a major role in life-long weight control. But you can only reduce fat if you know where to find it.

You can become a better judge of the foods you eat by learning to be a fat detective. In this chapter, you'll learn to read between the lines on product labels, navigate around the hype and misleading claims, and become a more educated low-fat consumer.

With a little practice, buying and eating lean will become second nature, and before you know it, the extra pounds will begin to disappear!

A Field Guide to Low-Fat Shopping

Your goal, first of all, should be to reduce the calories you get from fat to approximately 25 percent of your total caloric intake, a level many experts now feel is low enough to prevent the buildup of fatty deposits inside artery walls. This doesn't mean that every food you eat has to be 25 percent fat or less, but it does mean that 25 percent should be your overall average. This is why starchy foods, such as potatoes, bread, pasta, rice, and beans, can be so valuable. Because their calories are virtually fat-free, they can help to "balance out" the fat calories that you do eat.

Foods that you may think are low-fat starches, however, may not be if other high-fat ingredients have been added—so that's where the following "9 rule" can come in handy. There are 9 calories in 1 gram of fat. So, to calculate the percentage of fat calories in any food, check the label for grams of fat and calories per serving, then plug into this formula:

$$\frac{(grams\ of\ fat \times 9\ calories\ per\ gram)}{(total\ calories)} \times 100 = \begin{array}{l} percent\ of \\ calories\ from\ fat \end{array}$$

For example: A bag of potato chips says each 160-calorie serving has 10 grams of fat, so you multiply those 10 grams by 9 (90), then divide by total calories (160), which gives you 0.56. When you multiply by 100, the percentage of calories from fat equals roughly 56 percent.

Armed with that information, you can see that the 10 grams of fat in a single ounce of potato chips is no small peanuts.

So start counting percentages or start counting grams, but just start counting. Your health as well as your waistline will be glad you have.

Aisle by Aisle, from Thick to Thin

In the supermarket, a wide produce section takes first billing, followed by aisles and aisles of frozen foods. Then, wrapped around the perimeter, in a continuous band, are the deli, meat, dairy, and bakery sections. Once a bulging girdle of saturated fat, this outer strip has really tightened its belt. Today, with all the new light and leaner-than-ever products being stocked in the supermarket, it's among the hottest lanes for low-fat shopping. A special trip there— and to the packaged-goods aisles and ever-healthy produce section—will help you scout out the best buys (fat-wise) for your health and your waistline.

You'll see "read the label" many times as you read this chapter; that's because it's extremely important, especially in the beginning until you've identified the truly healthy foods. Remember, too, when percentage of fat means the percentage of fat calories—not to be confused with percentage of fat by weight, which is how some foods are labeled.

That said, here is an aisle-by-aisle guide.

Produce Section

Check Out:

Most fresh fruits and vegetables. Among nature's leanest foods.

Fresh herbs and aromatics. For flavor without fat, toss leaves of parsley, cilantro, and basil with your garden greens. Also, make use of fresh herbs, as well as leeks, onions, shallots, and garlic, in your cooking.

Lemons. Lemon rind or juice adds sparkle to meats, salads, or steamed vegetables.

Potatoes. Worth a special mention here; like pasta, beans and rice, these starchy (high-carbohydrate) spuds provide filling low-fat fare—the perfect counterbalance to moderately fatty foods.

Chestnuts. The one and only lean nut; just 5 percent fat (less than 1 gram per ounce).

Be Aware:

• Avocados and most nuts and seeds are low in saturated fat and high in polyunsaturated and heart-healthy mono-unsaturated oils. Use in moderation.

Pasta, Pasta Sauces, Rice, and Beans

Check Out:

All dried pasta, rice, and beans. With very little fat, these carbohydrates can replace fat calories in your diet. Be creative; instead of relegating them to the side-lines, try to plan your meals around them.

Canned beans and chick-peas packed in water. They have all the fat advantages of dried beans but save time in preparation.

Vegetarian beans with tomato sauce. Some contain only 9 percent fat.

Tomato sauce. Usually the leanest of pasta toppings.

Be Aware:

• Egg noodles do contain a small amount of cholesterol but are only about 12 percent fat.

• To reduce the sodium in canned beans or chick-peas, drain and soak in water before using.

• White pasta sauces, such as Alfredo and clam, are notoriously high in fat. Tipoff: Cream is the first or second ingredient on the label; cheese and butter also are featured prominently.

• Macaroni-and-cheese dinners usually do not contain low-fat cheese; to reduce the percentage of fat calories, add more pasta.

Dairy Case

Check Out:

1 percent low-fat and skim milk. The lean ones: "1 percent" milk can get 23 percent of its calories from fat; skim milk can range from 0 to 10 percent fat.

Buttermilk. Don't let its name mislead you; this cultured milk is only about 20 percent fat. Be aware, however, that buttermilk can be high in sodium.

Low-fat and nonfat yogurt. Low-fat or nonfat eating right out of the carton. Or drain yogurt overnight (using a sieve lined with cheesecloth or a coffee filter) and use as a cheese spread. A ¼-cup serving of nonfat yogurt cheese has no fat, compared to over 19 grams in an equal portion of regular cream cheese.

Reduced-fat sour cream. Reduced-fat versions have two-thirds the fat of the original. This amounts to 2 grams of fat per 2-tablespoon dollop, compared to 6 grams for regular.

Low-fat and (something new!) nonfat cottage cheese. Usually, no more than 11 percent fat; 0 for the nonfat version, which is available on the West Coast.

Fat-free mozzarella, American, and cheddar cheeses. Brand new on the market, these products have absolutely no fat.

"Lite" ricotta cheese. Part-skim one better: The lite version has 4 grams of fat per 4-ounce serving—one-fifth the amount in whole-milk ricotta and two-thirds less than the part-skim products.

Sapsago. A naturally low-fat (26 percent) grating cheese.

Light cheddar, Colby, and Swiss cheeses. In some cases, fat content is cut nearly to half of the regular version. Light cheddar carries about 5 to 6 grams of fat per ounce, compared to regular cheddar, which runs about 9 grams, for example.

Reduced-calorie or diet margarine. About half the fat and calories of regular margarine.

Any tub margarine. Always spreadable, it goes on thin so you get less fat on your bread.

Be Aware:

• To further reduce percentage of fat calories, serve cheese with a very low-fat cracker or whole-grain bread.

Cookies and Crackers

Check Out:

Matzo. Essentially fat-free.

Scandinavian crisp bread. From 0 to 1 gram of fat per slice, depending on variety.

Melba toast. Just 0.2 grams of fat per slice (about 10 percent).

Rice cakes and popcorn cakes. At most, rice cakes contain 0.3 grams of fat per "cake" (7 percent fat); popcorn cakes are usually fat-free.

Bread-stuffing cubes. They're dried, not fried like croutons; use in soups and salads.

Soda crackers. Tend to be lower in fat than most commonly used crackers, with 2 grams or less per ½-ounce serving (30 percent fat). Fat-free soda crackers should be available soon, if they're not already.

Fig bars, raisin biscuits, graham crackers. These old-time favorites fit today's low-fat diets, with under 3 grams of fat per ounce (usually less than 18 percent fat).

Be Aware:

• To reduce the percentage of fat calories consumed with a cracker snack, serve with all-fruit preserves, a nonfat yogurt cheese spread, or nonfat cheese.

Canned Goods

Check Out:

Cranberry sauce and applesauce. Flavorful meal accompaniments with no fat.

Water-packed vegetables and fruits in their own juices. If there's any fat in these products, it's not worth mentioning.

Cream-style corn. Surprise: just 1 gram of fat per ½ cup serving (from 9 to 11 percent fat).

Water-packed tuna. About 3 percent fat (less than

1 gram per 3-ounce serving) compared to 37 percent (7 grams per serving) for oil-packed.

Most noncream soups. Take your pick: chicken noodle, beef vegetable, split pea, tomato. All are in the 25 to 30 percent fat range—that's 6 grams of fat or less per bowl.

Be Aware:

• If you prefer the taste of oil-packed tuna, pour off excess oil, then rinse with cold water before using.
• Many canned goods are rather salty. Look for reduced-sodium versions whenever possible.

Oils, Vinegars, and Salad Dressings

Check Out:

Oil-free dressings. They contain no fat.

Dried salad-dressing mix. Allows you to blend your own dressing, using a minimum amount of oil.

Balsamic vinegar. Very flavorful and mild enough to stand on its own as a salad dressing.

No-stick sprays. Available with lecithin, corn oil, or olive oil; these sprays allow you to sauté vegetables and lean meats with a minimum amount of oil.

Light or cholesterol-free mayonnaise and mayonnaise-style dressing. Less than half the fat of regular mayonnaise, each teaspoon contains only about 1½ grams of fat.

Be Aware:

• Light vegetable oils are lighter in color and flavor, not lighter in fat or calories.
• Reduced-calorie dressings can also be low-fat, since lots of the calories in salad dressing come from oil. This isn't always the case, however. Check the label to see that it contains no more than 1 gram of fat per 1-tablespoon serving.
• Most vegetable oils are low in saturated fat and high in

polyunsaturated and heart-healthy monounsaturated fats. Use in moderation to replace saturated fats in your diet.
• Cut the percentage of fat calories in a "dressed" salad by adding legumes, potatoes, pasta or other low-fat or nonfat carbohydrates.
• A squeeze of a lemon is sometimes all you need to enhance the flavor of mixed greens.

Baking Needs and Dry Mixes

Check Out:

Evaporated skim milk. Substitute for cream in coffee or recipes.

Powdered skim milk. Use to thicken skim milk or as a nonfat alternative to coffee creamers.

Herbs and spices. If you're paring down your larder, be sure to stock your spice cabinet. A pinch of thyme or a grind of fresh black pepper goes a long way to maximize food flavor.

Butter-flavor granules. Made from defatted butter solids blended with starch, salt, and other flavorings, this product contains virtually no fat. Sprinkle on baked potatoes. Or dissolve some in hot water and use in place of melted butter to brush on fish, vegetables, or bread before grilling.

Fruit-flavored gelatin mix. Contains no fat.

Angel-food cake mix. This is a truly light cake with no fat. Top with fresh strawberry or raspberry puree for a heavenly and totally guilt-free dessert.

Be Aware:

• Sometimes the fat and calorie values stated on dry-mix labels reflect the content of the dry ingredients, not the final values of the prepared product. If you add eggs, milk, and/or oil in the preparation, the final fat scores could be considerably higher.
• Some mixes offer the option of "no-cholesterol preparation" (i.e., the use of egg whites instead of whole eggs,

skim milk instead of whole). This can modify fat content somewhat. Check the information on the back of the box.

Cereals

Check Out:

Most whole-grain, high-fiber cereals. Generally low in fat. Shredded-wheat biscuits are fat-free; bran flakes run about 5 percent fat (less than 1 gram per cup); oatmeal runs about 15 percent (2½ grams per cup), for example.

Be Aware:

• Cereals that contain nuts and seeds may be higher in fat than all-grain products, but they can still fall within healthy (under 25 percent fat) limits. Read the labels. (See the section on cereal on page 55.)

Baked Goods

Check Out:

Pita pockets, English muffins, and bagels. Your leanest sandwich partners or breakfast breads, with a mere trace of fat.

Most breads and rolls. Under 20 percent fat (1 to 2 grams per slice).

Fat-free, cholesterol-free cakes. Angel food is the obvious choice. But other fat-free versions of high-fat desserts are now on the market.

Be Aware:

• Bran, blueberry, and other cake-type muffins can be hidden sources of fat. Check labels.

Snack Foods

Check Out:

Popping corn. Popped at home with an air popper, it contains no fat.

Pretzels. From 0 to 8 percent fat, depending on brand. Try the unsalted variety.

Bite-sized rice snacks. Something new, similar to rice cakes, these seasoned bite-size snacks are about 25 percent fat.

"Lite" snacks. They're usually lower in fat. For example, lite corn chips are 33 percent fat, compared to 45 percent for the regular version. It's still important to check labels, however; one "Lite Air-Popped Popcorn" was 45 percent fat.

Be Aware:

• Some products labeled "lite" are lower in sodium, not lower in fat.
• Dry roasting peanuts doesn't save you many fat calories; in fact, they are about 79 percent fat (a whopping 38 grams per ½ cup).
• Caramel corn is less than 9 percent fat, but high in calories due to the candy coating.
• To give air-popped popcorn a buttery flavor, add butter-flavor no-stick spray, or any no-stick spray followed with a sprinkle of butter-flavor granules.

Deli Case

Check Out:

Chipped dried beef. Contains only 21 percent fat.

Extra-lean ham. About 32 percent fat (2 grams or less per 1-ounce slice).

Sliced turkey breast, chicken breast, and turkey ham (made from thighs). Generally, the leanest of the lunch meats, available with 26 percent fat or less—roughly 1 gram per slice.

Be Aware:

• A label touting that a product is largely fat-free can be misleading. Usually, that claim is based on the percentage of fat by weight, not by calories. The percentage of fat calories in turkey bologna labeled "82 percent fat-free/ 18 percent fat," for example, was in fact 75 percent fat— only slightly better than beef bologna, which runs about 80 percent fat.

• Chicken or turkey franks are not necessarily better than beef or pork hot dogs. The poultry products surveyed ran from 71 to 76 percent fat. By comparison, a lite beef frank and a "lite-and-lean" beef/pork frank chosen in the store at random were 75 percent and 64 percent fat, respectively.

• Moderately fat lunch meats containing 3 to 4 grams of fat per 1-ounce slice needn't be eliminated from your diet. Just limit yourself to two slices sandwiched in whole-grain bread to bring total fat calories in around 20 percent.

• Many lunch meats are high in salt. Buy reduced-sodium versions whenever possible.

• Deli salads—whether chicken, ham, or tuna—can have a whopping amount of fat calories buried in the mayonnaise dressing.

Frozen Foods

Check Out:

Fruit bars and pops and nonfat frozen yogurt. With these fat-free treats, there's no such thing as denial.

Tofutti lite, low-fat frozen yogurt, ice milk, and sherbet. Honorable mention goes to these frozen desserts; many come in under 20 percent fat.

Most vegetables and fruits. No cream sauces, just plain produce; they contain a negligible amount of fat.

Egg substitutes. Some have no fat, but check the labels.

Light frozen entrées. A far cry from the 1950s' TV dinners, today's leaner versions are available with under 25 percent fat—some under 15 percent. "Light" doesn't always mean right, however; you'll have to do the arithmetic to identify the lean ones. If you find your fingers freezing up on the calculator, use this rule of thumb: If a dinner or entrée contains less than 10 grams of fat, it's probably under 30 percent fat. (See the section on frozen dinners on page 49.)

Be Aware:

• Fish sticks and chicken breast patties or cutlets can often be hidden sources of fat.

Meat Case

Check Out:

Turkey breast. Undeniably, your leanest meat choice. Grilled, broiled, or roasted—and served without the skin—it's only 5 percent fat (less than 1 gram per 3½-ounce serving).

Chicken breasts and turkey thighs and drumsticks. Prepared and served as described above, they're about 20 to 21 percent fat (under 4 grams per serving).

Top round cut of veal. Under 3 grams of fat per 3-ounce serving (20 percent fat).

Pork tenderloin. A trimmed roast is just 26 percent fat (about 4 grams per 3-ounce serving).

The leanest beef cuts: top round, eye of round, round tip, and top sirloin. Trimmed of visible fat, they range from 24 to 33 percent fat (about 4 to 6 grams per 3-ounce serving).

Leg of lamb. Trimmed and roasted, it's about 35 percent fat (roughly 6 grams per 3-ounce serving).

Be Aware:

• A 3-ounce portion of meat is roughly the size of a deck of cards.
• Ground beef, chicken, or turkey can have excess fat. It's better to choose a lean cut of meat, trim it (and in the case of poultry, remove the skin), then grind it yourself.

Seafood Case

Check Out:

Most white-flesh fin fish. Haddock, flounder, and red snapper are among the leanest catches, at 7 to 12 percent fat (under 2 grams per 3-ounce serving).

Most shellfish. Shrimp, scallops, and crab run from 10 to 14 percent fat; lobster is just 3 percent. Please note that they do contain some cholesterol, however.

Be Aware:

• Fatty fish, such as salmon, mackerel, and halibut, are low in saturated fat and high in heart-healthy omega-3 fatty acids. Use with a carbohydrate source, such as rice or potatoes, to reduce overall percentage of fat in the meal.

• Rather than dunking lobster in melted butter, dissolve butter-flavor granules in hot water, then brush on before broiling.

How Lean Is Your Diet? Take This Quiz

Now that you know where the fat is, you can ask yourself how much fat you normally eat. One way to find the answer is to write down everything you eat each day and look up the fat content on labels and charts. But that could take a while. Here's the easy way. Take this quiz, developed at the Northwest Lipid Research Clinic at the University of Washington in Seattle. It will give you the average of your daily fat intake. Clinic researchers tested it on 222 people who also kept food records and found out that the fat score from the test generally matched up with fat contents computed from the food record.

For each question, circle the number of the answer that best describes the way you have been eating recently.

1. How may ounces of meat, fish or poultry do you usually eat per day? (Three ounces of meat, fish, or chicken is any *one* of the following: one regular hamburger, ½ chicken breast, one chicken leg [thigh and drumstick], one pork chop, or three slices of presliced lunch meat.)

  1. I do not eat meat, fish, or poultry.
  2. I eat 3 ounces or less.
  3. I eat 4 to 6 ounces.
  4. I eat 7 or more ounces.

2. How much cheese do you eat per week?

  1. I avoid cheese altogether.
  2. I use only low-fat cheese such as ricotta or diet or low-fat cottage cheese.
  3. I eat whole-milk cheese (such as cheddar, Swiss, or Monterey Jack) one or two times per week.
  4. I eat whole-milk cheese three or more times per week.

3. What type of milk do you use?

  1. I use only skim or 1 percent milk or don't use milk.
  2. I usually use skim milk or 1 percent milk but use others occasionally.
  3. I usually use 2 percent or whole milk.

4. How many egg yolks do you use per week?

  1. I avoid all egg yolk and/or use only the egg substitute.
  2. I eat one to two eggs per week.
  3. I eat three or more eggs per week.

5. How often do you usually eat lunch meat, hot dogs, corned beef, spareribs, sausage, bacon, braunschweiger, or liver?

  1. I do not eat any of these meats.
  2. I eat them about once per week.

3. I eat them about two to four times per week.
4. I eat more than four servings per week.

6. How many commercial baked goods and how much ice cream do you usually eat (examples: cake, cookies, coffee cake, sweet rolls, doughnuts, etc.)?
    1. I avoid commercial baked goods and ice cream.
    2. I eat commercial baked goods or ice cream once a week.
    3. I eat commercial baked goods or ice cream two to four times per week.
    4. I eat commercial baked goods or ice cream more than four times per week.

7. What is the main type of fat you cook with?
    1. I don't use fat in cooking.
    2. I use safflower oil, sunflower oil, corn oil, or soybean oil.
    3. I use olive oil, peanut oil, or margarine.
    4. I use shortening or bacon drippings.

8. How often do you eat snack foods such as chips, fries, or party crackers (Triscuits, Wheat Thins, Ritz, etc.)?
    1. I avoid these snack foods.
    2. I eat one serving of these snacks per week.
    3. I eat these snacks two to four times per week.
    4. I eat these snack foods more than four times per week.

9. What spread do you usually use on bread, vegetables, etc.
    1. I don't use any spreads.
    2. I use soft (tub) or diet margarine.
    3. I use stick margarine.
    4. I use butter.

To score: Add up the numbers from each of your answers. If you score 15 or less, that's a low-fat diet.

Anything higher than 18 can be considered high fat. If your number is too high, incorporate the 1 and 2 answers into your diet as much as you can. Note that you can get away with one or two 4s as your answer, but only if you balance them out with enough 1s.

Livestock Changes

Good news: Beef is getting leaner, according to revised U.S. Department of Agriculture (USDA) beef tables. Changes in cattle feed have some impact, but the real reason—at least according to the National Cattlemen's Association—is that butchers are now trimming off more fat, which cuts down its saturated fat and calories.

Meanwhile, Back at the Farm . . .

Chickens are getting fatter, reports the USDA. Although still relatively low in fat compared to red meat, today's chickens are bred to reach market weight in six to eight weeks—half the time it used to take. The result is a disproportionate increase in body fat. Advice: Most of this excess fat lies in and under the skin, and in pockets by the stomach, so remove it to ensure a healthier meal.

More Than One Way to Skin a Chicken

Contrary to popular belief, removing the skin from a chicken after cooking instead of before will not raise the fat content of the meat. "When the skin is left on during cooking, then you take it off and see the moist meat underneath, you might think it's fatty, but it's not," says registered dietitian Linda Dieleman of the University of Minnesota. "You're just seeing moisture—which makes the meat more flavorful. The fat that's in the skin stays there—it doesn't migrate into the meat. The skin simply helps hold in the moisture."

That tasty tip is backed up by a study comparing chickens with skin removed before cooking to chickens with skin removed after cooking. No difference in calories or fat content was found. If you remove the skin before cooking only to add butter or oil to moisten the meat, "you may end up with more fat than if you had baked it with the skin on," says Dieleman.

The Healthy Chef's Guide to Cooking Oils

There's only one thing you really need to know about cooking oils: They're all 100 percent fat—120 calories per measly tablespoon.

But oils can remain a part of your diet if you use them sparingly. So here's some information that will allow you to make the right choices about what oils to use, when to use them, and how to select flavorful oils that carry a lot of satisfaction in a single drop.

THE 8 BEST COOKING OILS ◆

	(%) SATURATED FAT	(%) MONOUNSATURATED FAT	(%) POLYUNSATURATED FAT
Canola	6	62	31
Safflower	9	12	78
Sunflower	11	20	69
Corn	13	25	62
Peanut	13	49	33
Olive	14	77	9
Soybean	15	24	61
Rice bran	19	42	38

6 FATS TO AVOID			◆
	(%) SATURATED FAT	(%) MONOUNSATURATED FAT	(%) POLYUNSATURATED FAT
Vegetable shortening	26	43	25
Cottonseed oil	27	19	54
Lard	41	47	12
Animal fat shortening	44	48	5
Palm oil	51	39	10
Coconut oil	77	6	2

The bottom line: The top eight oils in the table on the opposite page have the least saturated fat, and no cholesterol. Some of the bottom six in the table above are also cholesterol-free, but their high saturated-fat levels will help raise your blood cholesterol. (The percentages don't add up to 100 because there are small measures of other fatty acids that don't affect cholesterol.)

The table on page 48 will help you pick the right oil for various types of cooking.

How to Read an Olive Oil Label

They take olive oil very seriously in Europe—so seriously, in fact, that there are laws about how it must be classified and labeled. Since virtually all the olive oil sold in the United States is imported from Europe, you need to know what their terms mean before you decide which oil to buy.

Virgin. This oil is pressed (never chemically extracted) from the fruit and the pit. In U.S.–produced oils, which account for less than 3 percent of the olive oil sold in this country, "virgin" means the oil is from the first pressing. Neither virgin nor extra-virgin olive oil should be

THE BEST OIL FOR THE JOB ♦

OIL	SALADS	SAUCES	STIR-FRYING & SAUTÉING	FRYING	BAKING
Almond	♦	♦	♦	—	—
Avocado	♦	♦	—	—	—
Canola	♦	♦	♦	♦	♦
Corn	♦	♦	♦	♦	♦
Grapeseed	♦	♦	♦	♦	♦
Olive	♦	♦	♦	—	—
Peanut	♦	♦	♦	♦	♦
Rice bran	♦	♦	♦	♦	♦
Safflower	♦	♦	♦	♦	♦
Sesame	♦	♦	♦	—	—
Soy	♦	♦	♦	♦	♦
Sunflower	♦	♦	♦	♦	♦
Walnut	♦	♦	—	—	—

NOTE: Although avocado, olive, walnut, and sesame oils are more flavorful, they are less refined and break down in high heat. The other
oils are more refined and are stable even at high temperatures, making
them very versatile.

used for frying, baking, searing, or any other high-temper-
ature cooking. (Use the more refined "pure" grade described below instead.) They are excellent, however, for
cooked sauces, dressings, and light sautéing.

Extra-virgin. This is the top-quality, and most costly,
oil from the first pressing. Under Common Market regula-
tions, extra-virgin olive oil must have an acidity level of
less than 1 percent, and its taste, color, and aroma must
be judged "perfect" by official experts.

Pure. Refined and filtered to reduce acidity and
lighten both color and aroma, this oil will have a less
"olivey" taste. Because it is more refined, it can be used
for sautéing and stir-frying.

Refined. This is the U.S. term for second-pressed and
chemically refined olive oil. Similar to "pure."

Extra-light. This is a product designed especially for the American market, where we are just learning to like oils with flavor—extra-light is extra-refined, which gives it its pale color and mild flavor. Extra-light is neither a legal classification nor a description of an oil's content of fat and calories, which are the same as any pourable oil: 13 grams per tablespoon and 120 calories. Use as you would any highly refined oil such as corn or sunflower.

Pam and Her Sisters

Cooking oil sprays, such as Pam, have been available for several years. For the most part, they are very light and flavorless, and their chief advantage is convenience. They are easy to use, and it's hard to spritz on a whole lot. When you use them according to directions, you add only about 2 calories per serving. They are especially good for spraying muffin tins and cookie sheets, and many people use them as a shot of insurance in nonstick pans.

Aerosols have gotten a bad reputation with people who are concerned about the environment, so most of the manufacturers of cooking sprays have switched to propellants that are safer for the atmosphere. But there is still no getting around the fact that you have to be careful around the stove with anything that is under pressure in an aerosol can. Don't use them near heat; apply only to cold pans, and never spray them near a lit burner or into a hot pan or oven.

Hot Choices for Frozen Dinners
By Liz Applegate, Ph.D.

lecturer for the Nutrition Department at the University of California, Davis and a columnist for Runner's World *magazine.*

To most health-minded eaters, the term "nutritious frozen dinner" seems contradictory. Since their introduction more than 30 years ago, the meals that became famous as "TV dinners" have earned a (justified) reputation for being high in calories, fat, and sodium.

However, frozen dinners have changed for the better— which has paid off for the companies that make them, as well as for consumers. With the recent addition of dinner lines designed specifically for those seeking good nutrition as well as convenience, frozen meal sales have soared beyond the $4 billion mark. (Of course, the fact that many of us have microwave ovens and no time to cook is another big factor in their success.)

Nutrition-conscious folks can now find more than 100 frozen meals that are low in calories, fat, saturated fat, and sodium. These meals are under 300 calories each, less (sometimes much less) than 30 percent fat, and available at your grocery store. In fact, several frozen food companies, including ConAgra (Healthy Choice) and Stouffer's (Right Course), now boldly label their frozen meals with detailed information about fat and carbohydrate content to make comparisons easier for the consumer.

If you've given frozen dinners the cold shoulder, you may want to take another look. By reading labels carefully and adding one or more side dishes such as a salad, vegetable, or hunk of bread to round out the meal, you can enjoy a quick, low-fat, high-carbohydrate meal.

6 Ways to Master the Frozen Food Aisle

When you're browsing the frozen food aisle, keep in mind that one frozen dinner represents a complete meal. Therefore, your choice should fit reasonably into your low-fat, high-carbohydrate diet. If you select an entrée or dinner that is moderately high in fat and/or sodium, you'll need to adjust your other meals to ensure a balanced diet. Follow these guidelines to select the best frozen meals.

Calories

Frozen dinners and main dishes range in calories from

under 300 to over 1,200. Choose dinners or main dishes that contain from 250 to 400 calories, as they contribute about one-fifth of your daily calorie needs and allow you to round out your meal with a salad, vegetable, or serving of bread or cooked grain. Avoid those with more than 1,000 calories, as they contribute about half the daily calorie needs of most adults.

Fat

Everybody should limit fat consumption to less than 25 to 30 percent of caloric intake. (Many nutritionists recommend keeping your percentage of fat at closer to 20 percent of calories, or about 45 to 55 grams a day, depending on how much you eat. As a rule of thumb, a 300-calorie dinner should contain less than 10 grams of fat, and a 400-calorie dinner, no more than 13 grams of fat.

Read labels closely to figure fat content. Use the "9 rule" to compute fat calories. (See the guide to low-fat shopping on page 31.) The most detailed labels show not only the percentage of total fat calories, but also the amounts of saturated and polyunsaturated fat. Some dinners, like Stouffer's Right Course entrées, even show a bar graph comparing the nutritional content of their meals to general dietary guidelines.

Protein

A 300- to 400-calorie meal should provide at least 15 grams of protein, or about 25 percent of your daily protein requirement. Along with the rest of your daily meals and snacks, you should easily take in enough protein for good health. Frozen dinners range from under 10 grams to more than 35 grams of protein.

Most TV dinners contain beef, poultry, veal, or seafood, but manufacturers are introducing more vegetarian dinners and main dishes. Stouffer's vegetarian chili, for example, offers a great low-fat option for those who avoid meat. However, because some vegetarian-style meals fall short on protein, you may need to supplement your protein intake with a serving of a low-fat dairy product (milk, cheese, or yogurt) or a helping of beans.

Sodium

Notorious for their high sodium content, many frozen dinners contain more than 1,500 milligrams of sodium, making them off-limits for anyone on a salt-restricted diet. The minimum daily requirement for sodium is 500 milligrams, and the maximum recommended amount is 2,400 milligrams per day. To keep sodium intake in check, select items that contain less than 900 milligrams. Frozen dinners that are light on sodium include Healthy Choice, Stouffer's Right Course, and Le Menu Light Style. With a little supermarket savvy, you can find many selections that contain less than 600 milligrams of sodium.

Vitamins A and C

Let's face it: Frozen dinners are not known for outstanding vitamin and mineral content. In fact, it's often their major shortcoming. Many frozen dinners offer only small, overprocessed servings of vitamin- and mineral-depleted vegetables. But this seems to be changing, as some of the new frozen dinners contain larger portions of less-processed vegetables. Read package labels to select dinners that supply over 30 percent of the U.S. Recommended Daily Allowance for vitamins A and C.

To improve the nutrient content of an otherwise healthy low-fat, high-carbohydrate, high-protein dinner, add a side dish that will boost the meal's vitamin, mineral, and fiber content. Check the suggestions in the section on beefing up nutrition on page 54 for meal add-ons to round out your frozen dinners.

Cholesterol

Many frozen dinner lines rightfully claim to be low in cholesterol. Most contain much less than the recommended maximum of 300 milligrams per day, but you should continue to read labels just to make sure.

The Language of the Label

Best-selling frozen dinners often bear the words *light, lite, lean,* or *slim,* implying that the meal is reduced-calorie and low in fat. However, with the exception of *light,* these words have no specific meaning on food labels. According to the Food and Drug Administration, the term *light* is supposed to be used on products that contain one-third fewer calories than the original product. Yet labels frequently trumpet the word *light* and other health-oriented terms to hook the consumer. Don't be fooled. Look beyond the hype and read the nutrition labels.

If you do so, you'll realize that many of the so-called lean and light dinners are anything but low in fat. Weight Watchers Chicken Nuggets, for example, derives over 50 percent of its calories from fat, and Armour Dinner Classics Lite Salisbury Steak meal has more than 40 percent fat calories.

Fortunately, not all light dinners are high-fat, high-calorie items. To avoid being sucked in by misleading labels, simply read carefully, and stick to the "9 rule." You'll be healthier for your mathematical effort.

Best Buys in Frozen Meals

Even though you now know what to look for in a nutritious frozen dinner, the table on page 54, compiled by the editors of *Food & Nutrition* newsletter, can spare you the tedium of reading labels—to say nothing of the risk of frostbite.

BEST BUYS IN THE FREEZER   ◆

FOOD	CALORIES	CALORIES FROM FAT (%)
Armour Classics Lite		
Chicken Burgundy	210	9
Shrimp Creole	260	7
Budget Gourmet Light		
Breast of Chicken in Wine Sauce	250	18
Oriental Beef	290	28
Healthy Choice		
Chicken L'Orange	260	7
Chicken and Pasta Divan	310	4
Mesquite Chicken	310	6
Lean Cuisine		
Fiesta Chicken	250	22
Filet of Fish Divan	260	24
Le Menu Light Style		
Glazed Chicken Breast	270	20
Veal Marsala	260	21
Right Course		
Shrimp Primavera	240	26
Weight Watchers		
Beef Fajitas	270	23
Deluxe Combination Pizza	300	24

Beef Up Nutrition

Boost the carbohydrate, fiber, vitamin, and mineral content of your frozen dinner with these quick side dishes.

• Baked potato topped with steamed broccoli and nonfat plain yogurt
• Fresh fruit salad topped with low-fat vanilla yogurt
• Tossed garden salad with ½ cup canned kidney beans and vinaigrette dressing

• Whole-wheat pita bread spread with 1 ounce part-skim ricotta cheese
• Celery sticks filled with low-fat cottage cheese and topped with green onions

A Slow Stroll down the Cereal Aisle

Go down the cereal aisle of any supermarket, and you'll see that breakfast foods have grown up. The top shelf, at adult eye-level, is full of boxes luring us with promises of good health: high fiber, with multiple whole grains, brans, and dried fruit mixed in wild abandon. And their labels also boast about what they don't have: no sodium, no cholesterol, no added sugar.

No longer do we pick a cereal for the best collect-'em-all prizes or the sweetest, most candylike sugar jolt. Cereal is now serious.

But before you plunk down $3 or more for a "healthy" new cereal, you might want to consider some of the stalwart old stand-bys, like All-Bran, Raisin Bran, and that childhood staff of life, Cheerios. Not only do they stack up well nutritionally to many of the newcomers, they tend to be cheaper as well. And their very longevity means you can always find them in your store; some of the much-ballyhooed new brands disappear from the shelves after attracting only small, though devoted, corps of fans.

Still, most of the new "adult" cereals are good food, and they have interesting combinations of tastes and textures. And dietitians say the new high-fiber cereals are, for the most part, worth their price. That's good news, because cereal can take a major chunk out of your grocery budget.

So out of this array of cereals, how do you choose which are best for you?

"There's no one perfect cereal," cautions Pat Harper, a registered dietitian and spokesperson for the American Dietetic Association. "But a bowl of a good cereal is the best possible breakfast, much better than bacon and eggs, and certainly superior to doughnuts or coffee cakes. Almost all cereals are low in fat and deliver good measures of many vitamins and minerals. And now no one argues about the many benefits of eating enough fiber."

The Fiber Factor

Fiber sells a lot of cereal these days, but how much fiber should a high-fiber cereal deliver? "It depends on what you want, and what you eat for the rest of the day," says Philadelphia registered dietitian Molly Kellogg. "If you don't eat many whole grain breads, dried beans, or fruits and vegetables, then you'd want one of the really high-fiber brands that have 10 or more grams per serving. But if you eat plenty of these other foods as well, then you can choose a cereal that has 4 or 5 grams per serving.

"Diabetics and people who are more concerned about their cholesterol levels should look for soluble fiber, which you get from oat and rice bran," recommends Kellogg. "You don't need as much soluble fiber in a serving, because apparently it takes less to be effective. Eating oat or rice bran for breakfast, though, doesn't mean you can have a cheeseburger for lunch."

Psyllium, another kind of soluble fiber that is the base for laxatives such as Metamucil, also appears to have cholesterol-fighting powers. But it is currently added to only one cereal, Kellogg's Heartwise.

It's possible to select a cereal that packs both kinds of fiber, for instance Ralston's Multi-Bran and Fruit Muesli and Kellogg's Müeslix. Or, suggest both dietitians, you can alternate, eating one kind one day and another the next.

Mixing cereals is another option both dietitians mentioned, since some of the highest bran cereals are not noted for their palatability. Combining a few tablespoons of a very-high-fiber brand like Fiber One or All-Bran with something a bit tastier like one of the Common Sense or

Ralston cereals gives you the blessings of bran in a cereal that you can face happily in the morning.

Flabby Cereal?

The issue of palatability brings us to the next consideration in cereal, its fat content. For the most part, cereals that have 3 or fewer grams of fat per serving fall into the "acceptable" category, according to experts. (Presuming, of course, that you float your cereal in skim or 1 percent milk.)

How Much Are You Eating?

Which brings us to another important point about reading the information you'll find on the side of the box—the serving size. How much nutrition you're getting from a cereal depends, of course, on how much you eat. And most of us seem to eat more than the serving size on most cereal labels.

During a taste test, the amount eaten in a standard breakfast was weighed and measured. Surprise! For the most part, the women in the group put 2 ounces in their bowls (the serving size, on average, is about 1 ounce) while the men, and the real carbohydrate freaks, put in 3 ounces or more.

That means that you're probably eating more calories, fat, fiber, and sugar in a standard bowl than you may think from what it says on the box. That's not necessarily bad. But it is something to be aware of, especially if, like some of the tasters, you eat two or more bowls of cereal in the morning, or use it as a snack.

When it came to taste, the testers favored the multigrain and fruit combinations. Taste is a very subjective quality, though, and almost every cereal sampled had its supporters.

Surprisingly, some of the heartiest whole grains didn't

stand up well to milk, becoming limp and soggy fast. This seemed especially true of the flaked cereals. They stayed tasty, though. The rice cereals, on the other hand, kept their crispness in milk, but their flavor drowned.

What Else Is in That Box?

What else should you be looking for in a cereal, and which ingredients can you disregard? According to some experts, one of the major nutrients you can pick up at breakfast is iron. "Any cereal that provides 25 percent or more of the Recommended Dietary Allowance [RDA] for iron is a good one," says Pat Harper.

The sugar content of these high-fiber cereals varies greatly, from none to 13 grams. Generally, the brands with high sugar levels get it from the fruit they contain, not from added sweeteners. But you should read the label if you're concerned about sugar, looking for anything that ends in "-ose," like sucrose or fructose, as well as for honey and corn syrup. But neither Kellogg nor Harper believes that the sugar content of these cereals is a major issue.

"Five grams of sugar is about a teaspoon," says Harper. "That's an acceptable level, and I wouldn't worry about 7 or 8 grams in a cereal with fruit in it. Those aren't 'empty' sugar calories, since you get so many other nutrients. But more sugar than that does suggest the calories are getting higher without the nutrients rising, too."

Sodium is another cereal ingredient that concerns many people. But Kellogg thinks most of us shouldn't worry about it. "Cereal is just not a high-sodium food, even after you've put the milk, which adds about 65 milligrams, on it," she says. "Take one of the brands that is relatively high in sodium, like Cheerios. Even if a person eats 2 ounces of it, they're getting less than 700 milligrams of sodium. In the context of that being one meal out of three for the day, that's still a very moderate level."

Everyone is being urged to increase complex carbohydrates, and eating cereal is an excellent way to do this. Fifteen to 20 grams per serving is a good amount.

"Part of This Complete Breakfast"

Both dietitians gave recommendations on what to eat with a good cereal to make a great breakfast: "A vitamin C source, such as juice or fruit." That's because vitamin C greatly enhances the absorption of iron. That's especially important here, because the iron in cereal is less easily taken up by our body than the iron in red meat.

Most people put milk on their cereal, which is good, since you don't get much calcium from dry cereal. The milk brings that mineral up to about 15 percent of the RDA, say the dietitians.

But while these new high-fiber cereals are excellent foods, they won't work miracles with your health unless the rest of your diet is also pretty good.

"You shouldn't hitch your diet to just one good food," says Harper. "You can't expect a bowl or two of cereal, no matter how high-fiber it is, to counter a day's worth of poor food choices."

The Scoop on Cereal

Sitting down for a healthy crunch of high-fiber cereal in the morning may help you curb how many calories you take in the rest of the day, a study suggests.

Fourteen volunteers started off their morning with a bowl of one of five cereals ranging from low to high in fiber content. After 3½ hours, they were guided to a buffet where they were invited to graze on burgers, peanut butter, pickles, corn chips, and other munchies. Those who ate the highest-fiber cereal for breakfast ate about 45 calories less than the group's average at the buffet.

To follow up, the researchers gave another 19 volunteers one of two breakfast cereals, either very low or very high in fiber. As before, people who started their day with the high-fiber cereal ate fewer calories (an average of about 90 fewer) at lunch. Their combined calorie consumption—breakfast plus lunch—was also lower.

"Although this was only a short-term study, it suggests that a high-fiber diet like this, continued over the span of a year, could possibly result in a 10-pound weight loss," says researcher Allen S. Levine, Ph.D., of the Veterans Administration Medical Center in Minneapolis. People usually equate eating fiber with feeling full. Surprisingly, though, feeling full was not the reason the fiber eaters ate less. "Even though the people did not perceive they were stuffed, they still consumed less food," says Dr. Levine. This suggests that eating fiber may help you limit total calories without making you feel bloated.

Introducing Soy Fiber: Move Over, Oat Bran

Welcome a new entry into the dietary fiber arena. Soy fiber may now share the health turf with oat, wheat, corn, and rice bran, and others.

Its possible virtues, according to studies: It may reduce blood cholesterol in people with elevated levels, just like oat bran and other soluble fibers. It may improve glucose tolerance and insulin response in people with Type-II diabetes. And it seems to keep the bowel working at good speed, as wheat bran does, probably because it contains insoluble as well as soluble fiber.

The soy fiber in this research isn't exactly the same as soy bran, which uses the whole soybean hull. This soy fiber comes from only the inside of the hulls. It's available in two forms: one for baking and one for stirring into beverages.

While soy fiber may have some of the same health benefits as oat bran, it tastes different and reacts differently in cooking. Soy fiber smells and tastes nutty and toasty, and its texture is powdery, like flour. And soy fiber is a more concentrated source of dietary fiber than oat bran: It contains 2 to 3 grams of dietary fiber per teaspoon, compared to about ½ gram per teaspoon for oat bran.

"It appears to be a valuable addition to our current fiber arsenal," says Belinda Maness Smith, research dietitian with the metabolic research group at the University of Kentucky. "It may be especially useful to people who currently aren't getting enough fiber because of an aversion to conventional sources."

The studies with soy fiber used 25 grams per day. Smaller amounts may also be beneficial, but that hasn't been tested. Just bear in mind that you can get too much of a good thing: Experts recommend that you not exceed 35 grams of dietary fiber per day (total from all sources).

If you'd like to get cooking with soy fiber, try this rule of thumb: When baking, use ¼ cup of soy fiber with every cup of wheat flour in pancakes, waffles, muffins, quick breads, and pie crusts. Always add liquid to your recipe, equal to the amount of soy fiber used.

The recipe for Banana-Strawberry Whip on page 156 shows a tasty way you can use soy fiber in a beverage.

But Before You Abandon Bran . . .

You may have heard about the study that claims the benefits of oat bran are largely exaggerated. True, some claims made by manufacturers of oat bran cereals and other products about its miraculous cholesterol-lowering abilities are based more on poetic license by advertisers than on medical fact.

But in oat bran's defense, you should understand how this so-called debunking study was conducted. A report in

Rodale Press's *Men's Health Newsletter* reveals what the popular press failed to notice.

First, the study only had 16 participants (too few to make such grand conclusions)—all of them women, and all with cholesterol levels that were either low or well within the desirable range. In addition, the "high-fiber" oat bran diet they were fed got a whopping 35 percent of its calories from fat. And a high-fat diet raises cholesterol more than oat bran can lower it.

Yet, despite the fact the subjects had no tendency to high cholesterol, they still raised their levels of HDLs (good cholesterol) and lowered their LDLs (bad cholesterol) more than another group fed a lower-fat diet that didn't contain oat bran. Of course, the study's authors dismissed this, since the subjects' cholesterol levels didn't drop as significantly as those of participants in earlier, more scientific and objective studies. Ergo, the scary headlines.

Advice: Continue to eat oat bran regularly to lower cholesterol and help you lose weight, but with the understanding that it helps as part of an overall healthy diet that's high in fiber and low in fat. It's not a miracle cure for a lifetime of bad eating.

How Fiber Won't Work

There's a rumor going around that you can lose weight on ice cream or candy bars, as long as you send them down the hatch with some bran or celery. The claim is that the fiber will escort a large portion of the calories out the back door. In fact, this is a wild exaggeration. On a low-fiber diet, an average stool may contain 100 calories, and if you eat more fiber, it will contain about 110 calories—an insignificant difference.

Armed with that information, you should also be cautious of baked goods, such as certain commercial muffins that advertise that they're fiber-rich. A recent study of local oat bran muffins, conducted by the *New York Times* and the Center for Science in the Public Interest, uncovered one muffin bulging with 29 grams of fat (the equivalent of three single-serving bags of potato chips), and another weighing in at an incredible 824 calories! No amount of fiber could counteract the fat in a muffin like that! If you buy packaged baked goods, read the labels and make sure the fiber count is over 3 grams per serving and the fat and calorie count are modest.

Dietary Fat Makes Your Brain Thick

Here's another reason to turn down that cheesecake for dessert after lunch: Not only can fatty foods add to your fat deposits in the long run, they can also have a disastrous effect on your ability to concentrate in the short run.

During the long digestive process that follows a high-fat meal, blood tends to be diverted to the stomach and intestines, and away from the brain, explains Judith Wurtman, Ph.D., a research scientist in the Department of Brain and Cognitive Sciences at the Massachusetts Institute of Technology, and author of *Managing Your Mind and Mood through Food.* Mental processes are slowed, the mind is dulled, and the result is sloppy thinking, or no thinking at all—not exactly qualities that would help you advance up the career ladder.

To Burn More Calories, Eat Food You Love!

The mere sight and smell of meat raises the metabolism of dogs for about 40 minutes. If dogs can burn calories just thinking about food, what about us?

Researchers in Quebec tried to answer that question: Is it possible that the sight, smell, and taste of foods we like stimulate our body to burn more calories than when we're faced with bland, boring foods? The answer? A resounding yes!

The question came up when the researchers observed that rats fed through a tube into their stomachs gained more weight over 30 days than rats who were allowed to eat as much lab chow as they wanted. They guessed that the smell and taste of the food had stimulated the "thermic effect of feeding"—the amount of calories burned in digesting, absorbing, and storing the food.

To test their hypothesis, the researchers measured the thermic effect when people ate a tasty meal and also when they had similar food forced into their stomach through a nasal tube. Sure enough, good old eating burned more calories. In another human study, eating a palatable meal burned more calories than eating the same meal mashed together and dried up into a not-so-palatable biscuit.

In a follow-up rat study, rats fed food pellets mixed with delectable meat or pie fillings gained less weight in a month than rats fed plain, boring rat chow, even though they all ate the same amount of calories.

The bottom line seems to be that eating foods you like—in moderation—has a positive long-term benefit on weight loss. Chalk it up as one more scientific vote against the grapefruit diets of the world.

CHAPTER

3

FIGHT FLAB WITH FITNESS: GET UP, GET MOVING!

Defeat the Fat
By Phil Dunphy

physical therapist, exercise physiologist, and former owner of HEAR (Health through Exercise and Rehabilitation)

Do you know what the most popular machine at a health club is? It's not a Nautilus or Universal weight-lifting machine. It's not a StairMaster, a rowing machine, a Lifecycle, or a treadmill.

It's the scale.

I took a new employee along while giving a potential customer a tour of our place a while ago, and after it was over, he told me that I had been wasting my time for the final 10 minutes. "You didn't have to show him the weight room, the aerobic machines, or the testing area," he told me. "As soon as this guy saw those high-tech digital scales in the locker room, he was sold."

Unfortunately, that new employee was right. It's a religion. "Scale worship." People determine the value of a workout solely by weighing themselves before and after.

You can hear them in the locker room: "Hey! I had a great workout! I lost half a pound!"

No, they didn't!

Dehydration is not fat loss. That ½ pound was mostly water, and you'll gain it all back from the first ½ pound of fluids you drink later on. You have to! Your tissues need that fluid.

How can you lose ½ pound a day and still gain 5 pounds that week?

"Scale worship" is probably the biggest reason that people who start a weight-loss program give it up. They get frustrated because they're "losing" this water weight every day and yet they're still putting on pounds in the long run.

When people tell me that they're working out and gaining weight, I explain that there are two possible reasons why.

First, they're *not* really working out. I've seen people spend 2 hours in a club without getting much exercise. They lift weights with bad form, and they fail to maintain any activity long enough to burn fat. They don't understand the principles behind strength gain and fat loss, so they wind up wasting their time.

Second, they *are* really working out. Other people quit for the worst possible reason—they're not "physically educated" enough to realize that their program *is* working. They're lifting weights properly and they're engaging in good, long continuous bouts of aerobic exercise. But they quit because their "weight" doesn't change.

Sometimes they'll even say, "Yeah, I've lost an inch or two around my waist, but I can't lose any real weight, so what's the point?"

The point is that they lost fat but gained muscle. That's the best possible combination. Ready to turn your life—and your looks—around? Here's the secret of the fitness universe: It doesn't matter how much you weigh (within reasonable limits, of course) if your percentage of body fat is low.

The Right Way to Measure Fat

A scale only gives you one number—your total body weight—which is relatively meaningless without knowing how much of that total is lean body (muscle) weight and how much is fat.

Those figures are expressed as a percentage: the percentage of your weight that's fat, or your "percentage of body fat."

Some fat is necessary. Men need 3 to 6 percent body fat, women need 9 to 12 percent; that's your "essential fat." Anything above that is "storage fat"—the stuff that makes you look bad.

There are several ways to measure your body fat.

Hydrostatic weighing. This is the "gold standard." It requires that you get dunked in a specially designed tank, which enables a computer you're hooked up to to determine how much of you is fat and how much is not. Most people, of course, do not have access to such sophisticated (and expensive) equipment.

Electrical impedance. A small, hand-held device estimates your percentage of body fat by measuring electrical resistance in your skin. Its results can be affected by the amount of water in your system, and it doesn't work well if you're excessively fat or thin.

Skin fold test. A pair of calipers is used to actually "measure" the amount of fat you have by taking readings at several parts of your body and then taking the average of those readings. Very dependent on the skills of the tester.

The mirror-and-closet test. Let's be honest about body fat. You can see it and you can feel it. If you look better in a mirror, your program is working. If your pants are getting looser, it's working.

Sidestep the Scale

Unless you're trying to "make weight" for a prizefight, forget the scale. I don't even care if you actively measure your percentage of body fat. Like I said, if you use your pants and the evidence of your eyes as a guide, you'll know if you're losing fat.

Yes, I know all about the "new" medical studies with twins that found some people to be genetically predisposed to be heavy and others to be thin. It's a great excuse to be fat if you want to use it.

The big point here is that everyone—no matter what their genetic makeup—will lower their percentage of body fat if they eat less fat and do more continuous exercise.

Some people do have a genetic "edge" that helps them see results fast; others take a longer time to trim down. But everyone can trim down. You can do it. You just have to want to do it.

Been sitting around for a long time? Start walking.

Work your way up to ½ hour a day. If you're already working out, keep it up! You're doing great!

Exercises That Burn More Fat

Want to burn more fat? Use more of your body. You burn more fat with an exercise that works your arms and legs than with one that just works your legs. You burn more fat when you exercise standing up than when sitting down because you're also carrying your body weight.

Those simple rules form the basis of this "fat-burning rating" of machines you might find at the nearest health club, gym, or YMCA. Here they are, from the best fat burners to the least effective.

Nordic Ski Machine/VersaClimber. These two are tied for first place. Both machines keep you vertical and really work your arms and legs. Excellent fat burn. The VersaClimber tends to appeal more to elite athletes.

StairMaster. This machine gives you good intensive exercise where you carry your own weight, but some types are better than others. Older models that have rotating sets of stairs like an escalator are best because you have to actually lift your legs to keep pace. Newer models have pedals, but there are two different types. One has an "independent step" system, where the pedals don't influence each other as you simulate that stair-climbing motion.

In some models, one pedal goes up automatically as you press the other one down. That's no good. You're not working half the time. And that makes this type much less effective at burning fat.

You probably can't control which type will be available, but you can maximize your workout on any of them by selecting the "manual control" setting and then picking a level you can maintain for 30 to 45 minutes.

Avoid those fun-type programs with rapid changes; you spend most of your time trying to maintain your balance. And once you get going, don't hold onto the rails;

let your arms hang by your sides or swing them as if you were power walking.

Also, if you drape yourself over the front of the machine with it set at a high level, you are wasting your time.

Treadmill. You're standing, which is what you want. Swing your arms and raise the incline level for a little extra work.

Rowing machine. Better than a bike because you're using your arms and your legs, but very few people can pace themselves slowly enough so that they can last for 30 to 45 minutes. It's also the machine on which people tend to have the worst form.

Keep your back straight; don't lean forward. Your arms should always come straight back and forward. Time your strokes so that your knees are down and out of the way when your arms pass over them. You should never have to raise your arms to clear your knees.

Bikes. People love to ride them because they can sit down. If you're already that tired, how much fat do you think you're going to burn? And if you lean forward to make it look like you're racing, you'll burn even less.

Try to find a recumbent bike where you're lying down instead. They're better fat burners because their relationship with gravity makes you work harder.

No club, gym, or YMCA? You can buy the cheaper, smaller home versions of this equipment, but most people never use it. Generally, you can't make any adjustments on these things, and taller people may not be able to stand up straight while exercising. (If you can't stand up straight, don't use it.)

If you want to try one, buy it on your credit card so you can be sure and get your money back if it doesn't work out.

The Absolute Best Place to Lose Fat

It's the mall. No kidding. You can get a great workout in a mall. Start by walking from one end to the other to warm up. Then pick a spot where there are two escalators side by side, or a set of stairs. Walk up and down them (you should never just ride an escalator; it's like having free time on a StairMaster—use it!) for half an hour, and then walk from one end of the mall to the other again to cool down.

It's a great workout, and bad weather won't hold you back. Same thing with an airport. To kill time between planes, walk from one end of an airport to the other. If you're in Chicago or Atlanta, you'll get an Olympic-level workout. And no matter which airport you're in, power-walking to kill time not only burns fat, it also loosens you up enough that you won't feel stiff after you get off the plane.

Stuck in a hotel in a strange town? Climb up and down the stairwell for an hour. In fact, you should take the stairs every chance you get. It builds up your endurance and it gets your body used to exercise.

Increase your everyday activity. Walk more. Take the steps. You'll gradually raise your BMR—your Basal Metabolic Rate. And that will help you burn fat more efficently when you exercise.

Hang On for 45

Unless you are a serious high-intensity athlete, it takes time for your body to mobilize its fat stores when you exercise. For 99 percent of the population, the first 20 minutes of any continuous exercise is set-up time, during which you burn mostly sugar for energy. But if you keep moving, you burn fat after that.

So, 30 minutes of continuous exercise is necessary to burn some fat. Go for another 15 minutes—a total of 45 minutes of continuous motion—and you may burn twice as much fat as if you had stopped at 30.

Should you go for an hour, then? I don't think so. My advice for a good, long-term fat-loss plan is to shoot for 45 minutes of continuous movement three or four times a week instead of an hour once or twice a week.

Two reasons why: One, you increase your risk of injury

when you continue longer than 45 minutes, due to the repetitive motion involved and the greater chance of serious fatigue.

Two, working out more frequently raises your BMR and makes you a more efficient fat-burner.

Do 45 continuous minutes three or four times a week and you'll drop a pound of fat a week. You'll look great. And more important, you'll begin to feel great, too.

Lift Weight to Lose Weight

Dieters who add circuit weight training—a program in which you alternate short periods of weight lifting and aerobic exercise—to their fitness regimen lose more fat and less muscle than aerobicizers or people who don't exercise at all. Mary Ellen Sweeney, M.D., of Emory University, told a meeting of the North American Association for the Study of Obesity that women who used weights and exercise machines had 85 percent of the weight loss as fat, compared to 72 percent fat loss in walkers and nonexercisers.

This is not to knock walking for weight loss, says Dr. Sweeney, but to point out that some forms of exercise are better than others at improving proportions of body fat to muscle.

Weight training, by the way, isn't only for the muscle-bound. One study at Tufts University showed that ordinary people in their eighties and nineties benefited from weight training dramatically, increasing both strength and muscle mass.

Find a Fitness Center That Fits

Ads for fitness clubs sizzle with rippling muscles and tight stomachs. They make it seem so glamorous.

Reality isn't always so pretty, however. Some health centers are plagued with dirt, crowds, and unqualified instructors. And then there are the take-the-money-and-run schemes.

It doesn't have to be that way. Some health clubs offer great trainers, great machines, and a variety of exercises to keep you hopping in any weather. Fitness teacher, philosopher, and merchandiser Jack LaLanne and the Better Business Bureau have helpful hints for finding the workout facility you want.

Round up the candidates. Commercial health clubs aren't the only places to work out. Colleges sometimes open their gyms to the community. Some hospitals sponsor fitness centers. And, of course, there's your local YMCA.

Critique the atmosphere. Pay a trial visit at the time you want to exercise. "Question as many members as you can," advises LaLanne. "Ask them if they like the place, and what they don't like about it." Is it crowded? Are the lines too long when your workout time is short? Do you feel comfortable with the regulars? What kind of place do you want? Bare-bones bodybuilding, or comfort and class, glass and chrome?

Consider the price. Have a price range in mind, and check to see what your membership includes. Some clubs have varying price structures based on access to certain equipment, length of membership, and hours of operation.

Keep your fitness goals in mind. If it's aerobic action you need, make sure there is a variety of options on hand. Dance classes, pools, treadmills, and exercycles will do the trick. Consider, too, what you'll actually do. Why pay extra for racquetball courts, pools, weight machines, and saunas when all you really want is an aerobics class?

Read the report card. "There are so many fly-by-nights these days," says LaLanne. Ask for a reliability report from the local Better Business Bureau.

Read the fine print. "Don't sign any long contracts

until you find out their validity," says LaLanne. Don't be pressured into signing anything right away. Take the contract home and read it over. Is everything promised written down? Is the club bonded so that if the place goes under you can claim a refund?

Try a trial plan. "A lifetime health-club membership may seem like a bargain, but not when you consider that the membership is for the lifetime of the club, not necessarily the lifetime of the member," *Consumers Digest* cautions. They advise that you purchase only one-year or short-term memberships to protect you if the club suddenly closes or you lose interest in it.

Scrutinize the club premises. "Cleanliness is paramount," says LaLanne. Also make sure the equipment is up-to-date and working.

Check for quality qualifications. Instructors should have bachelor's degrees in exercise physiology or similar fields, LaLanne says, or certification by the American College of Sports Medicine.

Make sure the instructors guide you. To LaLanne, it's essential that the instructors make sure the members are reaching their goals. "The instructors should get to know the members," he says. In one study, researchers found that successful exercise programs have trained instructors who can devise the right program for you and encourage you to stick with it.

Consider convenience. When are they open? Can you fit regular visits into your schedule? If it's too much of a drag to get there, you won't stick with it. Walking is easier to cram into busy schedules—you can do it just about any place, any time.

Stroll into Super Shape

Good news, walkers! You can get more body-sculpting power from the same amount of walking if you use the "healthwalking techniques" developed by Howard Jake Jacobson, owner and director of the Sparta Fitness Center in New York State and author of *Racewalk to Fitness.*

"My method is really the racewalking technique, minus the competition," says Jacobson. "But if I call it racewalking, people get scared."

The technique tightens your tummy, buttocks, arms, and legs more than regular walking does. "When you straighten your leg as you plant your heel, you actually use more muscles (hamstrings, buttocks muscles) than when you run," explains Jacobson. "This takes the same effort, but you get use of additional muscles. The result is more toning of the affected muscles."

To shape your calf muscles, he suggests you learn to push off with your toes instead of the ball of your foot because you work your calf muscles harder that way.

And if you pump your arms like a sprinter—bending your arms at the elbow and swinging them forward aggressively (being careful not to raise your shoulders)—you can tone your upper arms and back muscles, Jacobson adds.

Fine-Tune Your Technique

Prevention magazine challenged six of the top walking coaches in America: "If you could offer one tip to help eight million readers improve their ability to walk for health and fitness, what would that tip be?" Their different answers were surprising, but all of their tips are geared to helping you get more out of a walk: more speed, more power, more stamina, more relaxation. If you're walking for fitness, and you're ready to put a little more zip into your workout, try these techniques from the experts.

Find your proper stride length, Anne Kashiwa, director of the Rockport Walk Leader Program and author of *Fitness Walking for Women*, says. "I notice in my clinics and classes that many people try to go faster by taking exaggerated steps. Then they tire too quickly." To find your proper stride length, stand, lean forward at the ankle (like a ski jumper in midair), let yourself fall forward, and catch yourself by extending one leg. That's your natural stride length. "If you step too far out, you'll actually begin to lean backward. You're trying to travel in one direction but leaning in the opposite direction. That's counterproductive. It is much better to take more steps using your natural stride than to take fewer exaggerated strides."

Bend your arms, says Casey Meyers, author of *Aerobic Walking* and lecturer at the Aerobic Center in Dallas. "One thing that helps a walker progress from, say, 15-minute miles to 13-, 12- or even 11-minute miles is the bent-arm swing technique. The long, extended arm is one thing that impedes a walker from going faster. The arm and leg have natural swings that correspond to each other. If the arm is extended, it acts as a long pendulum that swings more slowly and holds you back."

You can test this yourself. Walk briskly with your arms bent at the elbow (at a right angle), swinging back and forth. After a few minutes, deliberately extend your arms. It feels like you're dropping an anchor! Keep your arms extended and swinging for a few minutes, then bend them at the elbow again. You'll feel an extra boost in speed.

"On the forward swing, your arm should cross your body slightly, but your hand should not be higher than the top of your breast," says Meyers. "On the back swing, the hand should go back no farther than the center of your hip."

Relax your upper body, says Steven Jonas, M.D., triathlete, author of several books, and coauthor of *PaceWalking: The Balanced Way to Aerobic Health.* "It's important to keep your shoulders down when you swing your arms. When you hunch your shoulders in an effort to go faster, you get tension across your chest, your shoulders, and the back of your neck. That's counterproductive to the relaxing effect walking can bring to you. And it doesn't make you go faster!

"You'll have to continuously remind yourself, 'Drop those shoulders!' until it's second nature."

Become more flexible around the hips and torso, says Bob Carlson, championship racewalker and coauthor of *Healthwalk.* "Most people have lost the hip and torso flexibility they were born with. And rigidity there interferes with efficient walking.

"I recommend that people straighten their knees when the knee comes under the body, as in racewalking, so that the body rides on the bone, not the muscle. This pushes the leg up into the hip socket and promotes flexibility in the hip area. Pointing your feet straight ahead and landing your feet directly in front of each other (like walking a tightrope) helps rotate the hips horizontally around the spinal column, another area where people are rigid. Doing 'windmills' (rotating the arms backward, like doing the backstroke) helps create flexibility in the upper body. Stretching exercises for the hips and waist can help, too."

Use the psoas for more muscle power, say David and Deena Balboa, coauthors of *Walk for Life* and co-directors of the Walking Center of New York City. "To walk with more power and better balance and posture, imagine that your legs begin 2 inches above your navel," says David, a sports psychotherapist. "In a sense, they do. The psoas muscles, located just below the rib cage, attach to the lower spine, the pelvis, and the femur bone in the thigh, and are like a bridge between your upper and lower body. By sensing that the action of your legs really begins with the psoas, you'll develop a fluid, gliding walking style— more like skating along than lifting the leg and trudging. Let your hips swing freely. You'll feel a more powerful stride because you'll be using more muscle power. In working with our clients, Deena and I have found this single tip to have the greatest impact on people's ability to walk with power and grace."

These Shoes Are Made for Walking

If you're walking your weight off, treat your feet to a good pair of walking shoes. It could prevent de agony of de feet.

If you're on the prowl for some walking shoes, here are some shopping tips on how to find the perfect pair.

• The best time to shop for shoes is late in the day. The simple biological truth is that your feet tend to swell as the day goes on, especially if you've been standing on them all day.

• When you're trying on walking shoes, bring a pair of socks with you that you plan to wear when you walk. Comfortable, thick socks or those that wick away moisture and sweat are usually available at most shoe stores.

• Buyer beware: Just because you are a size 7 doesn't mean that a size 7 walking shoe will fit. You may require a shoe larger or wider than your normal casual shoe.

• Make sure you have an adequate toe box (the top portion of the shoe). To judge, place your thumb at the tip of your longest toe. The space should be about ½ to ¾ inch to the tip of the shoe. Then stand on your tip-toes. The back of the shoe shouldn't come off your heels.

• Take your time. Don't be afraid to walk around the store a couple of times. These are shoes that will be seeing a lot of action, so give them some basic training first.

• If you're very heavy or prone to aching feet, you may have to wear a shock-absorbing running shoe to cushion the impact of your weight when you walk. Ask your doctor or podiatrist to recommend a good pair.

Gear Up Your Exercise Cycle

If you're gearing up for weight loss through stationary biking, here's how to get the most mileage from the experience.

• Make sure your bike fits. If it doesn't, you won't feel comfortable. In fact, you could hurt yourself. Start with the saddle, women's biggest complaint about bikes. Check the width by sitting on it. The saddle should support your pelvic bones, not dig into your flesh. If the saddle does dig into you, have a bike dealer show you some wider ones. If you're using a gym bike and can't readily change the seat, cushion it with a foam or sheepskin pad.
• Check saddle height. If you push the pedal all the way down with the ball of your foot, your knee should be slightly flexed.
• Adjust the cant—the angle of the saddle. (Even on the cheapest of bikes you should be able to adjust the seat.) If the front is too high, it can cause discomfort. Remedy: Adjust the saddle so the front is parallel to the top tube or tipped slightly down.
• Once the seat is right, check the handlebars. Set the height and angle so that when you hold them, you lean only slightly forward. Place just a little weight on your arms. That way, you're not likely to strain your lower back.
• Take it easy, especially at first. Set the bike's resistance low enough that you can pedal comfortably. Too much resistance can inflame tendons and hurt ligaments and cartilage in your knee.

A good beginner's workout goes like this: First do 40 revolutions per minute (rpm)—10 revolutions every 15 seconds for 3 to 5 minutes. Then move to the main part of the workout. Accelerate to 60 rpm: one revolution per second. An easy way to estimate this is to count 1,001, 1,002, with each revolution. Try to keep cycling for a total of 20 minutes.

When you've done your time, cool down by pedaling at a lower speed and resistance for 3 to 5 minutes. For your last minute, slow to 40 rpm.

You may need to modify the intensity of this regimen, of course, to maintain your target heart rate or to ensure comfort. In any event, you should end this workout after the 20 to 25 minutes are up or you feel you've done enough, whichever comes first.

When you do finish, walk around the room a few minutes. And don't shower or bathe for at least 10 minutes after you stop exercising. You may unduly stress your heart.

• Change hand positions during workouts. Doing so changes the position of your back and arms, reducing soreness. Periodically stand up and pedal for 30 seconds, too. This relieves saddle pressure and stretches your legs.

• When the beginner's routine doesn't tire you, try tougher workouts. Within a few weeks, you can raise your sights to at least 70 percent, but no more than 80 percent, of your maximum heart rate. Get there by adding more resistance, riding for at least 2 minutes, and checking your pulse.

Keep adjusting resistance until you can stay at your new target heart rate for a 20- to 25-minute workout. By adding 1 to 2 minutes to every other session, you can eventually work up to 45 minutes a day, six days a week.

On the seventh day, rest. Cycling six days a week is enough.

• Make sure the bike has a weighted flywheel. That's the smooth-running wheel with a friction belt that regulates resistance. Bikes that regulate resistance by increasing pressure on the wheel, or those with caliper brakes, tend to be jerky and no fun to pedal.

• Get your money's worth. For a decent new stationary bike with basic features, expect to pay $125 to $500. High-tech bikes cost more: $1,200 to $2,100. Some of them have displays that estimate the calories you burn, count your rpms, take you through a preprogrammed warm-up and cool-down, and let you race against a computer-generated opponent.

• Try variations. Some bikes exercise not just your legs but your arms and torso, too. As you pedal, you move the swinging handlebars back and forth with your arms. With such dual-action bikes, air resistance generates the workload, so in these models no flywheel is necessary. And in most models, the resistance stirs the air enough to give you a pleasant breeze. If your legs get tired, you can pedal less and let your arms do the work. Price: $400 to $700.

• If, because of hip or back problems, you can't use a standard indoor bicycle, you may still be able to cycle. On a recumbent exercise bike, you pedal sitting, as if you were in a chair. There's a backrest to support you, and your legs go in front of rather than underneath you. Prices start at $200.

If you have back trouble, check with your doctor before you try either the dual-action or recumbent models. And don't use them if they hurt.

Row, Row, Row to Slimness

Like dual-action bikes, rowing machines shape up not just leg muscles but also the chest, back, trunk, and arms. Here's how to get maximum benefit from any rowing machine.

• Get expert help. Start your rowing career with a back evaluation, preferably from your family doctor or back specialist. He can prescribe exercises to stretch and strengthen your lower back muscles. Have an instructor show you proper rowing technique, too. It's easy to learn.

• Adjust the footrest to a comfortable angle. Otherwise,

the footrest can flex your ankles uncomfortably and prevent you from making a full stroke.

• Use the comfort lover's training schedule. To prevent back injury, begin your rowing regimen with low resistance and a minimum number of strokes. If you have arthritis, start with 20 strokes a day. Add 20 strokes a week, building up to 100. Use rowing as part of an overall fitness program.

If you don't have arthritis, warm up by rowing 12 strokes a minute for 5 minutes. Since rowing works out all the major muscle groups, you may tire quickly. Don't feel bad if the warmup is all you can do at first. Let your heart rate, or what feels comfortable, guide you. Increase your rowing gradually, adding 10 percent a week to your number of strokes per minute. Ultimately, aim for 22 to 24 strokes per minute. When you can row for 20 minutes, add more power to your workouts. Every 2 or 3 minutes, for instance, pull harder for ten strokes. Or alternate periods of hard rowing with easy rowing. Later, increase the time and intensity of your workout still more. And at the end of each workout, cool down with some slow stretching.

• Buy quality. Avoid rowing machines that use a knob tightened on a wheel to provide resistance. Such machines are too jerky. Two types of units are worth considering.

Hydraulic cylinder rowers, quiet and small enough to sit in a corner, are the most popular at-home models. The higher on the rowing arm you clamp the cylinder, the greater the resistance. Price: $129 to $400.

Straight-pull rowers cost more. Some come with an electronic speedometer, stroke counter, timer, calorie counter, and like the high-tech bikes, a computer-generated rower you can race against. A flywheel braked by a fan, belt, or motor provides resistance. Price: $650 and up. Whatever machine you buy, make sure the seat rides on ball bearings, not plastic. And look for joints that are welded together, not bolted. Bolts and plastic wear out quickly.

Step Up Your Workouts

Bench-stepping, which consists of stepping up and down on a bench or sturdy box, is an excellent and inexpensive aerobic conditioner that requires little space. Frederic Goss, Ph.D., and his colleagues at the University of Pittsburgh report that bench-steppers can reach 90 percent of their maximum heart rate during a workout. A routine consisting of making 20 steps per minute burns about 10 calories per minute, while a more vigorous 30-step workout burns about 16 calories per minute. Add 2-pound hand weights and you increase caloric burn by about 14 percent.

Innovative Exercise:
Boogie Down to Size

Their workouts used to take them miles apart. He'd jog left on a Saturday morning, she'd walk right. There was a lot of distance in their marriage in those days, too.

Then they tried something one weekend on a friend's advice. They skipped their Saturday morning workouts and went dancing that night, instead. And guess what? They've been burning calories cheek to cheek every Saturday night ever since. This tale is a composite of stories we hear all the time: Moving feet draw people closer.

"It's the ultimate togetherness workout," says Phil Martin, a lecturer and dance instructor at California State University, Long Beach. "You move in a physical harmony that works toward an emotional harmony. You also tend to bring back a lot of fond memories. The dance floor can be a great place to give a tiring relationship a second wind." Not just the heartstrings get pulled by the likes of a good fox-trot, however: The heart itself gets a loving tug.

"Studies show that steps such as the cha-cha, polka, samba, Viennese waltz, and East- and West-Coast swing easily can raise the average person's heart rate enough to achieve an aerobic-conditioning effect," Martin says. "You tend not to realize it, though, because you're having too much fun."

Aha! Fun. That word seems to have gotten pushed aside in recent years by all the treadmills, gut busters, rowing machines, and stationary bikes. "No pain, no gain" has been our fitness credo. And yet very little fitness has been gained.

"Surveys show that fewer than 15 percent of Americans have been successful at sticking to the kind of three-workouts-a-week schedule currently recommended for good cardiovascular health," says Bryant A. Stamford, Ph.D., director of the Health Promotion and Wellness Center at the University of Louisville and coauthor of *Fitness without Exercise.* "We need more fitness activities that let people have a good time. That encourage them to be creative rather than compulsive. That encourage them to communicate and not just perspire."

Don't Just Exercise, Celebrate!

Lee Walker, M.D., wholeheartedly agrees. The 75-year-old physician from LaFollette, Tennessee, traded his sweat suit for a pair of blue jeans years ago. Dr. Walker, you see, is a square dancer, and has been for about 50 years. "It can be a heck of a good workout but also a heck of a good time," he says.

"Studies using pedometers have shown most square dancers cover about 5 miles in a single night," says Stan Burdick, coeditor of *American Square Dance* magazine.

Nice. And especially nice considering the social mileage that gets covered. "People bring their whole families," Dr. Walker says. "Children and grandparents alike take part. It's exercise but it's also a form of celebration. Not a lot of other fitness activities can say that."

No, with most other fitness pursuits you're either alone or you're competing. But when you dance, you're cooperating, Martin says. "The goal in dancing is to work with rather than against another person, and it can have very positive emotional spillovers."

Take Andy and Michelle Feldman, for example, who not only fell head over heels for each other at one of Martin's dance classes but decided to keep the ball rolling by spending their honeymoon at one of his week-long dance camps. "Dancing definitely revs up the romantic side," Martin says.

Not all dancers fire up as easily as the Feldmans, however. Sometimes people need a little push to get started. Consider the case of 47-year-old George from California, for example, who used to joke that, sure, he'd go dancing—if he could take his portable TV! But George's wife Diana finally broke him down one weekend, and bingo: Now George is the guy up there asking the band for "just one more" every Saturday night, brow sweating, shirttail on the loose. And he's also the guy now jogging or playing volleyball at least three times a week.

"The dancing made me feel young—young enough to be a little bothered at how strenuous it seemed," George says. "It was a nice way to get kicked in the rear to get back in shape."

"I see it a lot," Martin says. "People get reawakened to the joy of physical movement, and it inspires them to want to do more. Many people even start making positive changes in their diet."

Happy Feet Make Happy People

Maybe the most remarkable benefits to be gained by dance have to do with that area well above the feet—the mind. Researchers from the departments of psychology and dance at Reed College decided to study just that. They assigned a group of 133 college students to either a sports class (which taught kayaking, fencing, and basketball), an academic class (with instruction in biology, religion, and American literature), or a dance class. The students were asked to respond to a 20-item self-evaluation both before and after their participation as a way of measuring the influence of the class on their sense of well-being.

Here's what the authors reported about the study's results: "Relative to the academic students, dancers characterized themselves at the end of the class as more creative, happier, more secure, stronger, more confident, more relaxed, more exhilarated, more motivated, healthier, and more competent."

And how did the dancers compare to the sports participants? "Dancers felt significantly more creative, confident, relaxed, excited, motivated, healthy, intelligent, and energetic."

Theories vary on exactly why dance has such mood-elevating powers, but central among them is that dance emphasizes expression and creativity more than competition. And that may have a very liberating effect.

Swing Your Calories Away

Is it an exaggeration to call ballroom dancing "great exercise"?

Hardly. Tests by the Department of Human Movement and Recreation Studies at the University of West Australia have found that a robust rumba can be as aerobically demanding as running. That a torrid tango can raise the heart rate higher than a hot game of squash. That even just a well-done waltz can court the cardiovascular system as aggressively as a brisk walk. "Dancing several times per week can make a valuable training contribution...to persons seeking to...enhance their level of fitness," the researchers conclude.

And it can be a great way to step away from some unwanted body fat, too. Researchers from the Department of Physical Education at San Diego State University recently found that a 12-week program of low-impact aerobic dance resulted in body fat losses averaging an impressive 7 pounds per participant. Plus there were no injuries and no dropouts! Sessions lasted 45 minutes and were conducted three days a week. Then, too, if you're out dancing on evenings you might otherwise be home snacking, you're getting a double weight-loss benefit.

Which steps are capable of caressing the heart best?

Based on a study of 45 dance-class students at California State University at Long Beach, the styles noted below raised people's heart rates to within their "target zones"—the level of exertion needed to produce an aerobic conditioning effect. "Any dance can be performed with different intensities, however," says Martin. "The amount of exercise afforded ultimately depends as much on the dancer as the dance."

So go slow or go wild, depending on what you're trying to achieve. And keep in mind that you tend to burn more calories, not fewer, the better you get at any given step. Some dances more than others can help you achieve your target heart rate (60 percent or above estimated maximum heart rate). Of those doing the East Coast swing (i.e., jitterbug, lindy, or bop), about 95 percent hit their target heart rate, with 91 perecnt for the polka, 80 percent for the Viennese waltz, 75 percent for the samba, and 44 percent for the cha-cha. Other good aerobic workouts include the mambo and square dancing.

Runners: Green Is Less Mean

"If a horse can't eat it, I don't want to play on it," was Philadelphia Phillie Dick Allen's initial comment on the then-new artificial surface, Astroturf, some decades ago. And the ace home-run hitter's opinion was definitely on the right track, say biomechanics experts at Lehigh University in Bethlehem, Pennsylvania. Of all surfaces tested, good old natural grass was found to cause the least stress on the joints of a runner who covered 15 to 20 miles a week. Running on asphalt produced the worst shocks to the system, they found. But the researchers fell short of declaring grass number one, because of the danger of falling into an occasional divot. Instead, they recommend professional-style polyurethane tracks, which are kind to your joints and free of gopher holes.

Try Some Mini-Motivators

Whether you're a skier, a stair climber, or a stationary cyclist, there are a few gadgets and gimmicks that can help you keep at it.

• Check your form in a mirror. Watch your upright stance on a ski machine, monitor your knee/toe alignment on a stair climber, or just admire your ever-shapelier self in a wall-mounted mirror.
• Add some motivational posters, if they reflect your true convictions. Some Rome-wasn't-built-in-a-day-type posters may help you keep gliding, climbing, and cycling week after week. Hang them near the machine where you can't possibly miss them.
• Let the sun shine in—but not on—your workout. Sunshine will brighten up your workout area and probably your workout. But don't overdo it. Placing your machines directly in the sun's rays can turn you into a solar-heat collector.
• Try a portable heart-rate monitor. A pulse monitor that clips to your ear or finger costs $60 to $150; a heart monitor goes for about $150 to $300. Ask at a sporting goods store. A monitor makes it easy to check your exertion level at a glance and gives you I-can-do-it incentive.
• Position your exercise equipment in the coolest spot in your house. A room that's comfortable for lounging may

seem like a sauna while you're biking. Temperatures in the low 60's are best.

• Choose the right music. Listening to music can motivate you, but a too-dominant rock-type beat can compete with the steady pace you're striving to maintain. Try show tunes or the Brandenburg Concertos instead.

Special Advice for Beginners

Follow your heart or how you feel. Depending on your temperament, let one of two indicators guide the intensity of your workout. If you'd like an objective measure of how hard to cycle or row or participate in any fitness activity, go by your heart rate, which is measured in beats per minute. You can estimate your maximum heart rate by subtracting your age from 220. When you exercise, you should reach 50 to 70 percent of that rate initially, and eventually work up to 75 to 80 percent.

You'll probably have to slow down a bit to check your pulse. Don't slow down for long, though. Take your pulse on the artery that runs along your right wrist toward your thumb. Using the fingertips of your left hand, you should find your pulse easily. To estimate your heart rate, take your pulse for 10 seconds and multiply by six. That will give you total number of heartbeats per minute.

For workouts on ski machines and stair climbers, your target rate should be about 60 percent of maximum. To figure your 60-percent-of-maximum target rate, subtract your age from 220, and multiply that number by 0.6. It's just too easy to start working too hard on these machines, overstressing heart and lungs. Besides, if you start sweating heavily too early in your workout, your muscles will fatigue and you won't last long enough to enjoy serious fat-searing results.

If you don't want to bother with the numbers, you can simply do what feels comfortable. You should be breathing

◆

deeply and rapidly, as if you've climbed a flight of stairs. But you should always have enough breath to talk while you exercise. (As in any exercise, if you feel abnormal heartbeats, pain, dizziness, or other distress, you should stop the workout and see a doctor.)

Use a fan, or fan yourself with a wind-load bike or rowing machine. The breeze simulates conditions outdoors, drying perspiration before it builds up too much. A fan can double the time you spend working out.

Drink water before, during, and after each session. That can help prevent dehydration and heat stress. Heat makes you tire faster, and dehydration can be dangerous.

Put your exercise machine someplace conspicuous. If it's in your living room, you're more likely to stick to your regimen than if it's tucked away somewhere.

Pick a workout time when you normally don't have conflicting duties. That way, excuses for skipping a workout will be just about impossible to find.

Hypertensives Beware:
Caffeine and Exercise Don't Mix

If you're prone to high blood pressure, you might want to make sure you're decaffeinated before you hit the jogging path. Exercise normally causes blood pressure to rise slightly. But a cup of coffee before you start may intensify the surge, according to a study.

Thirty-four men aged 21 to 35 years who had normal blood pressure participated in the study. Before straddling exercise bikes, they took either an amount of caffeine equivalent to about 2 to 3 cups of brewed coffee, or a placebo (blank pill). After a period of rest, they rode at various levels of intensity. The experiment was repeated another day with the caffeine-takers switching to the placebo and vice versa.

The caffeine combined with exercise temporarily produced high blood pressure in 44 percent of the subjects tested—more than twice the number who showed this short-term rise in blood pressure from exercise alone. What's more, caffeine caused blood pressure to continue increasing throughout moderate to maximum exercise.

"We were surprised to see the effects of caffeine on blood pressure at all stages of exercise," says William R. Lovallo, Ph.D., associate research career scientist at the Veterans Affairs Medical Center in Oklahoma City. Usually, moderate to heavy exercise dilates blood vessels, boosting blood flow to your muscles and keeping blood pressure from rising too high.

The study was done on men with normal blood pressure, but it's possible the results may hold true for people with high blood pressure, says Dr. Lovallo. "With caffeine increasing blood pressure in moderate to maximum exercise stages, people with hypertension, or at risk for developing it, may want to limit their caffeine on days they plan to exercise."

Exercise: It's Not Just for Weight Loss Anymore

In addition to helping you stay in good physical shape, a lifelong habit of regular exercise may also keep you on your toes mentally, according to a study at Scripps College in Claremont, California.

In a series of tests, researchers there compared 62 highly active people aged 55 to 91 with an equal number of nonexercisers of the same age. The purpose was to see if being physically active has a positive effect on cognitive (thinking) skills as we grow older. The high-exercise group included older athletes of all shapes and stripes, with serious walkers, weight lifters, and marathon runners among them. Two 1½-hour sessions of tests assessed reasoning, reaction time, and memory. The researchers found that the high-exercise group performed significantly better in all reasoning tests, in all reaction-time tests, and in two of the three memory tests.

Louise Clarkson-Smith, Ph.D., who conducted the research with Alan A. Hartley, Ph.D., says, "I think this study strongly suggests that exercise is important in preserving our mental abilities as we get older."

Dr. Clarkson-Smith says that it is not likely that the high-exercise group was healthier to start with and so performed better. Her analysis ruled out health as a significant factor.

Some researchers speculate that the decline of mental and physical energy as we age may be linked to a decline in our central nervous system's efficiency, which may be affected by circulation to the brain. So physical exercise, which is known to improve the efficiency of circulation in older people, might help keep the cognitive skills fresh.

Diet Burnout?
Let Speedwalking Reignite You!

Lately, does it feel like you walk all day and don't get anywhere—in terms of weight loss, that is? Sure, going for distance—and consistency—sets you on the right track. And during the first few months of walking regularly, the inches may have just slipped away. But now that your body's accustomed to the workout, you may find your progress has reached a standstill. What happened?

Maybe you've walked yourself right onto a weight-loss plateau. The calories you're exercising away—combined with your habitual diet—are now just enough to maintain your new lower weight. But don't worry. With a little extra effort, you can sashay right off that plateau and resume progress to your ideal weight.

How? By supplementing your regular walking program with speedwalking! Not to be confused with racewalking with its unusual hip moves, speedwalking is simply walking at a quicker pace. Studies show that as your pace quickens, your calorie burn quickens even faster. Many fitness walkers cover a mile in about 15 minutes (a speed of 4 mph), burning roughly 365 calories per hour, or about 90 calories a mile.

But bump your speed up to a 12-minute mile (5 mph) and your calorie burn goes all the way to about 585 for the same hour—or about 117 calories a mile. That's a bonus of 27 calories a mile!

Those 220 extra calories you're burning each day can translate to a weight loss of about 15 pounds in less than a year. And you'll be burning the same number of calories as a runner going the same 5 mph speed.

The big difference, though, is that you'll be losing weight with much less chance of strain or injury.

"In running, you leave the ground on every stride. And you land with three to four times your body weight," says James M. Rippe, M.D., director of the Exercise Physiology and Nutrition Laboratory at the University of Massachusetts Medical School. "With walking, one foot is always in contact with the ground. So you land with only 1 to 1½ times your body weight."

A Few Pointers to Get You Going

Bet you never thought you'd be learning to walk again. But, as with any exercise, there are important lessons you should learn before you set out to speedwalk.

First, before you even take a step, remember that warming up is important in keeping your walking safe. When you speedwalk, you get a good upper-body workout you may miss when strolling or running. To make sure that your shoulders, arms, and legs are warmed up, walk at a slow to comfortable pace for 5 to 10 minutes before your workout. You may stretch after warming up, or you may wait until after your workout.

Second, you'll want to ease into your speedwalking routine gradually. Don't assume that just because you're a veteran walker, you can go from 4 mph to 5 mph in only one day.

Incorporate speedwalking slowly into your walking program. At about the midpoint in your daily walk, when your muscles are warm, pick up your pace. You should feel that you're walking faster, but not so fast that you're gasping for breath. Maintain the faster pace for no more than 1 minute. Do the same the following two days. On day four, extend the time you're speedwalking to 2 minutes. Hold at 2 minutes for a few days. Then add on another minute of speedwalking. And so on. If at any time you experience strange or painful symptoms, slow down immediately. Your body may not be as eager to speedwalk as your mind.

The biggest mistake you can make is to walk too fast, or maintain an accelerated pace for too long. Do either, and you're sure to experience painful cramps.

But progress slowly and you will probably be able to increase the time of your speedwalking to 10, 15, or even 30 minutes. But be patient—this will happen over a couple of months, not weeks.

Only when you're able to speedwalk comfortably for at least 10 minutes at a stretch should you experiment with increasing your pace another notch. And if you're more than 15 to 20 pounds over your ideal weight, please don't do any speedwalking. Instead, maintain your regular walking program until you reach a lighter weight. Then try speedwalking to knock off those last 10 or 15 pounds.

Here are some additional tips from walking expert

Viisha Sedlak, president of the American Racewalk Association.

Go solo. Sure, it's more fun walking with company. But when you're a beginning speedwalker, take a couple of walks by yourself. You're more likely to pay attention to your own body signals when you're walking alone. Then, when you're used to speedwalking, take friends along.

Set your sights a little higher, mentally and literally. Walking with your head down can cause stress in the lower back, Sedlak says. Try to focus straight ahead while walking.

Walk tall. Watch your basic posture, too. Your shoulders should be down and open, not hunched. "Think of opening the chest and dropping the shoulders so there's no tension," Sedlak says. "Then lift the ribs and upper torso off the hips so that the diaphragm and abdominal muscles are free to move."

Forget the fancy footwork. As the song goes, just put one foot in front of the other. Walk with your feet straight in front of you; walking pigeon-toed or duckfooted can lead to painful knee problems. Also, check the way your feet are landing. You should land on your heel and roll off your toe with each stride. You may experience initial pain in the muscle at the front of your shin. That's because it's natural to keep your foot flexed throughout your stride and forget to roll off your toe. Then, you're using that muscle far more than normal. And that can lead to inflammation.

If you find yourself with a sore shin muscle, back off from your training program. Treat your leg to ice, rest, and elevation, Sedlak says. Also, during and after your walk, try this stretch: Press the toe of your sneaker into the ground and lean forward with your shin. You'll get right to the muscle in question.

Let 'er roll. Now walk. That's all there is to it.

And the great thing about walking is it's one of the

few weight-bearing activities you can do every day. So get out there and walk as often as you can. But keep this in mind when you're scheduling your walking time on a day-to-day basis: 20 minutes is the length of time it takes to begin burning fat. Tom R. Thomas, Ph.D., a University of Missouri exercise physiologist, explains: "Fat's usually going to come from adipose tissue and it has to travel to muscle. So there's a time lag when you start exercising."

That means it's best to walk for at least ½ hour so you have at least 10 minutes of high fat utilization, he says. If you don't have that much time to walk each day, by all means get going for the time you do have. "Calories are calories," Dr. Thomas adds. "It's nice to burn fat calories, but it's good to burn any calories." Walking is a good fat-burner, according to a study Dr. Thomas conducted that compared it with cycling, skiing, and rowing. In that study, subjects performed the four different exercises at the same heart rate for each type of exercise. Walking fared better than the non-weight-bearing exercises (cycling and rowing) with 40 percent of total energy expenditure coming from fat.

So if it's slimming you're after, speedwalking is a great way to go. And it may give your walking program the kick it needs to get you over that weight-loss plateau.

CHAPTER

4

THE MIND/BODY CONNECTION: HOW YOUR BRAIN HELPS SLIM YOUR BODY

Lifelong Weight Control from the Inside Out

For Marsha Blair, losing weight was a 15-year-long losing proposition. She struggled with one diet after another and watched helplessly as the weight inevitably crept back on.

"I hated being fat and I was miserable because I just couldn't seem to do anything about it," she says. "I felt totally out of control."

Having exhausted every diet plan and program imaginable—and still 125 pounds from her goal weight—Blair decided it was time to accept her fate.

"I realized I was spending my whole life fighting this weight battle. I wasn't happy with myself or my life. I kept thinking that some day, when I lost the weight, I'd be able to do all the things I wanted to do. In effect," she says, "I was postponing living."

It was at this point that Blair took a bold new stance: She made up her mind that, even if she couldn't be thin, she could be happy. She stopped badgering and criticizing herself about her weight problem. She shopped for new clothes and makeup, reviving her pride in the way she looked. She started treating herself with respect.

What happened after that?

Believe it or not, Blair (who, along with her husband, Scott, won *Prevention* magazine's Husband/Wife Body Makeover Contest) succeeded at losing 112 pounds. She's kept it off, too, for almost two years now.

Accept Yourself

"It's as if you have to love it before you can lose it," says eating disorders expert Emily Fox Kales, Ph.D., of McLean Hospital in Boston. "Liking yourself 'as is' enables you to care enough to take steps to improve your body physically."

Dr. Kales finds that many people who can't accept themselves overweight organize their lives around the day when they'll be thin. "I see overweight women who live in baggy clothes because they feel undeserving of nice clothes. It's a form of self-flagellation," she says.

So many of us—women in particular—are critical of our bodies, expecting perfection. Joyce Nash, Ph.D., a clinical psychologist and author of *Maximize Your Body Potential,* believes that this perfectionism often stands in the way of successful weight loss. "I have patients who feel that their eating behavior and bodies have to be flawless." The problem with perfectionist standards is that you set yourself up for failure.

"People who always strive to reach the ideal constantly feel they should do better," says Dr. Nash. No matter what they've achieved, it's not enough. They'll chastise themselves for falling a half pound short of their weekly goal rather than acknowledging the fact that they're making progress. Or they'll quit dieting altogether just because they happened to give in to one irresistible craving.

To make matters worse, "each time [a dieter] loses then regains weight, she loses a little more self-respect and gains greater feelings of shame and inadequacy," adds Thomas Wadden, Ph.D., co-director of the University of Pennsylvania Obesity Research Clinic.

Overwhelmed with feelings of worthlessness—and driven by her own negative thoughts—she gets caught in a vicious circle of failure. Too often, then, weight control becomes her nemesis. She'll deny herself her favorite treats and sentence herself to high-intensity, do-or-die workouts. Sometimes she'll force herself into uncomfortably tight clothes, thinking that will motivate her to stop eating. The odds that anyone can peel pounds permanently with this approach may be pretty slim. Chances are, you'll be so miserable, you'll look to food to soothe yourself, Dr. Kales warns.

Build a Better Body Image

Building self-esteem is the often overlooked but critical first step to any weight-loss program, explains *Prevention* adviser Kelly Brownell, Ph.D., co-director of the University of Pennsylvania Obesity Research Clinic. If you care about yourself, you'll be inclined to exercise regularly because it makes you feel good. You'll be willing to embrace a healthful, slimming diet, because your body thrives on it. And you can recover from the occasional binge—and get right back on course—because you forgive yourself. In short, you'll be in control.

To get started, here are a few body-image building exercises.

Think of yourself as attractive, now. Take pride in your appearance. Treat yourself to a manicure. Try a flattering new hairstyle. Buy yourself a new dress sized to fit you comfortably, now. What's important is that you develop a positive attitude about the way you look at your present weight.

As a case in point, noted weight-control expert Susan Wooley, Ph.D., at the University of Cincinnati College of Medicine, describes an attractive client who complained about acquaintances criticizing her weight. Dr. Wooley asked the client to go through one day imagining herself as the most beautiful person on earth.

Having followed Dr. Wooley's advice, the woman reported that total strangers complimented her on her appearance. Dr. Wooley's point is that if you hold yourself in high esteem, others will treat you in ways that continue to make you feel good about yourself.

Be nice to yourself. Buy yourself flowers, tickets to the theater, or a book you've been wanting. Don't wait until you've lost the weight to start living.

Focus on your strengths. Do you have a good sense

of humor? Are you skilled at your job? Do you have a knack for parenting? Do you care about social causes? Is creativity your forte? Do you have a network of very good friends? Are you romantic? Usually, the things you're good at are the things you enjoy doing. So make it a point to work at building your strengths every day—and remind yourself of your accomplishments.

Stop feeling guilty about your weight problem. "We try to unhook people from the notion that being overweight is a mortal sin," says Dr. Kales.

Be realistic about what you can achieve. "Accept the things about you that you cannot change," says Dr. Nash. Genetics and metabolism are important contributors to weight problems. If you've been 75 pounds overweight for 15 years, for example, you may have to settle for a goal weight that's somewhat higher than what the "ideal weight charts" specify.

Set small, manageable goals. Start by choosing one or two small positive changes you can make today that you'll be successful at. They may be as simple as taking a 10-minute walk at lunch or eating an apple instead of a doughnut on your morning coffee break. At the end of the day, acknowledge your accomplishments, no matter how small they may be.

Stop gearing your life around food and your weight. As Dr. Nash puts it, "Life is not about weight control. It's about having a commitment beyond yourself— raising a family, contributing to your community, doing a good job."

Start exercising now. A moderate program of aerobic exercise (like a brisk walk at least every other day) is a way of being good to yourself—and not just because it burns calories. One theory about why exercise increases the likelihood of losing weight and keeping it off is that it boosts your mood and self-esteem. Dr. Kales believes that exercise also can give you a sense of control that, in turn, improves your self-concept. Bean Robinson, Ph.D., a Minneapolis-St. Paul–based psychologist, is another proponent of using exercise as a body-image builder. Those who are self-conscious about exercising in front of others should go about it more privately, she says. Take a walk in the park. Or buy indoor exercise equipment like a stationary bicycle.

Dr. Robinson also advises that you abandon silly notions about exercise clothing. "A lot of 'large' people have rules about what they can and can't wear. Many won't wear shorts, for instance." Try to free yourself from these ideas.

Your Personal Pep Talk

How you talk to yourself throughout the day can also have a tremendous impact on your self-image—and the success of your weight-loss program. Whether you know it or not, you talk to yourself all the time, not necessarily consciously or out loud. If you see a chocolate cake on the counter, for instance, your body isn't automatically drawn to it. In deciding whether to have a piece, you might say to yourself, "I've had a tough day. I deserve this." Or, "I've been dieting all week and haven't lost a pound, so I may as well eat it."

What's your next likely course of action? Probably cake-eating. But what might happen if instead you said to yourself, "I've had a bad day, but it won't solve anything if I eat cake. It won't make me feel any better." This kind of self-talk may well prevent you from eating.

The point is that self-talk plays an important role in determining how you'll act and how you feel about yourself. If your self-talk is negative and defeating, you may likely engage in self-destructive behavior like binge eating or nibbling when you're not even hungry. On the other hand, if your self-talk is positive, you can often prevent inappropriate eating and feeling bad about yourself.

Here are some suggestions from the experts about how to make your self-talk more positive.

Develop an awareness of your negative, self-defeating thoughts. Each time you overeat or feel you've strayed from your goals, reflect on your thoughts before, during, and after you ate. (It helps some people to keep a thought diary.) Even better, try to get in touch with yourself before the fact; when you feel like eating, stop and think about what's going through your head. Let's say you find yourself reaching into a bag of cookies while you're sitting in a traffic jam on your way home from work. You may find yourself thinking something like, "This will make me feel better." Or, "I've eaten three cookies, so I may as well eat the whole bag." If you have trouble getting in touch with your self-statements, say to yourself, "I'm acting as if. . .," and complete the sentence. You might say, "I'm acting as if dinner is 3 hours away." Or, "I'm acting as if this will make the traffic jam go away."

Analyze your thoughts. Ask yourself if they're rational, true, or helpful. In the case of the traffic jam, ask if it's really true that you can't wait until dinner. (After all, are you going to die if you don't eat the cookies?) Will eating the cookies really make the traffic jam break up? Will you really feel better after having eaten a whole bag of cookies? In the long run, will a mere three cookies make any big difference in your weight?

Challenge your thoughts. Come up with more positive, helpful self-statements. For example, "Of course, I can wait until dinner; if I wait, the hunger may pass." Or, "Eating will not solve the problem." As for the classic, "I may as well eat the whole bag," challenge it with "Three cookies won't make me gain weight, but eating the whole bag might."

Give yourself credit. Instead of obsessing about the one day out of an entire week that you overate, focus on the six that went just fine.

Stop "catastrophizing." Instead of saying, "If I don't lose all this weight before my class reunion, I won't go," say to yourself, "I'll do my best. If I lose even a few pounds, I'll feel better."

Don't make excuses or rationalize. Challenge thoughts like, "There's no way I can cut back with the holidays coming." Or, "I deserve to eat it since I've been so good." Instead say, "It's hard to watch what I eat when I go out, but I can plan ahead." Or, "I deserve to celebrate, but I'll buy myself something other than food."

Avoid "never" and "forever" statements. How realistic is it to think that you'll never eat another candy bar or that you'll exercise every day for the rest of your life? Give yourself permission to deviate; no one can be perfect all the time. Marsha Blair, loser of 112 pounds, says she thinks she failed on many diets because she couldn't have certain foods. "It just made me want them more," she says. Now she gives herself the option of eating treats, which makes them less attractive. On a recent trip, she allowed herself dessert each night. But she doesn't do that every day.

Stop using food as a "Band-Aid." Blair admits she used to eat when she was tired, bored, or angry. Now, when she feels like eating, she talks to herself, asking if she's truly hungry or if something else is bothering her. It makes sense: If you're not really hungry, you should try to figure out an alternative to eating, like taking a hot bath or going for a walk—something that will really make you feel better.

Change your "hot" thoughts to "cool" ones. When you're in a tempting food-related situation, you can have two types of thoughts, says Dr. Nash. "Hot" thoughts focus on how good something would taste and how awful it would be if you couldn't have it. "Cool" thoughts, on the other hand, are more distanced, analytical ones that distract you from temptation. For instance, "It's not really worth it to eat that candy when I've made so much progress. Besides, I know what it tastes like and I can have it again some other day." Sometimes it helps to wait for 10 minutes and see how you feel.

Avoid using negative, punitive words to describe yourself or your actions. "Stupid," "bad," and "cheat" are all no-nos. They only get in the way of feeling good about yourself and are usually way off base. After all, are you really a bad person just because you ate an extra piece of bread? Isn't "cheating" rather an extreme accusation if you go off your food plan? (Think about what it means to really cheat, say, on taxes or a school exam.) A more positive self-statement would be, "So I ate an extra slice of bread at dinner. I'll be more careful about my eating tomorrow."

Don't create self-fulfilling prophecies. If you tell yourself you'll always be overweight and that you're a failure, how can you ever hope for success? One woman who kept a self-statement diary found herself saying, "I'll never lose weight. I lack self- discipline." She challenged it with, "I can lose weight if I don't overeat." She acknowledged that the self-discipline accusation wasn't entirely true: "I complete my obligations on time." Then she rewarded herself with a trip to the library. Another time her negative self-statement was, "I am fat and unattractive," which she countered with, "I can be more attractive by wearing makeup and a nice dress."

Being more accepting of your body and yourself in general doesn't mean resignation to bad eating habits or inaction. Since you need your body, Dr. Nash stresses the need to take care of it. She sums it up nicely with, "You are not your body, but you are not separate from it, either."

She feels that learning to feel good about yourself increases the likelihood that you'll be able to maintain new eating and exercise habits for a lifetime.

Manage Your Moods without Food
By Marilee Goldberg, Ph.D.
psychotherapist and specialist on weight and well-being

Would you like a foolproof way to make all your unpleasant emotions go away?

Most of us would. And I wish I could give it to you, but I can't because life just doesn't work that way. Still, you can learn how to manage your moods—to stop them from controlling you, to stop them from fueling binges, and to feel better in the long run. This is one of the foundations of effective weight management.

One of the keys, paradoxically, is to stop avoiding emotions. Just as gauges on the dashboard of a car signal when you're running low on gas or oil, feelings give you valuable signals about your needs. Ignoring either signal can get you into trouble. And if you block negative feelings such as inadequacy and anger, you also block positive feelings such as joy and love.

Not only that, attempts to make "bad" feelings go away usually backfire. For instance, when we try to comfort ourselves with food or alcohol, we can gain weight. And when we try to avoid painful feelings such as rejection by avoiding social situations, we may end up feeling lonely and isolated. These avoidance strategies might make us feel better in the short run, but they hurt us in the long run because they keep us from facing our real problems and solving them. And to top it all off, we feel inadequate, ashamed, helpless, or frustrated for having these feelings in the first place.

There is a better way. For starters, it's a good idea to accept all emotions, pleasant or not. Occasionally, a person might cry when discussing something that is emotionally charged. But such breakdowns can often reveal what hasn't been working in your life. That makes all emotions useful because you can begin to correct the problem once you realize what's going wrong. Here are some examples of problem-solving approaches to emotions.

Figure out what's up. When you feel a strong urge to eat and you're not even hungry, there's probably something eating at you. Ask yourself what it is. If the only answer you can come up with is, "I feel bad," work at getting more specific. For example, are you anxious, bored, lonely, lethargic, restless, nervous, hopeless, frustrated, disappointed, or insecure? The answer could give you some new choices about what you can do to feel something more desirable.

"If you are aware only that you feel bad when visiting relatives, you are left with the option of either not visiting them, or visiting them and enduring the bad feelings," write Leslie Cameron-Bandler and Michael Lebeau in *The Emotional Hostage.* "However, if you are aware that you are feeling, say, bored, you also have the choice of doing something to make the visit more interesting. If you are feeling irritated, you can request that the person stop their offensive behavior."

Learn from your emotions. No matter how unpleasant, odious, or awful an emotion seems to be, it can be useful if you respond to it as an opportunity to learn about yourself. So instead of focusing on the discomfort and feeling sorry for yourself, take the feelings as signals of what is amiss in how you're currently doing things.

For example, frustration can deepen into despair if you take it as evidence of your inability to accomplish what you want. But it can be useful when you realize it means you're still working toward something even though you're not getting results now. So if you still want to accomplish your goal, you need to gather more information, get new instructions, or try a different approach.

A feeling of emptiness can be helpful if you take it as a signal that you're open and ready to start something new.

Now, no one can make a prescription for each emotion. One mood can mean different things for different people. In general, though, one great way to get at what's bothering you, deep down, is to ask yourself a few questions. Here are a some good ones to start with.

"What am I saying to myself that contributed to the mood?"

"How did I contribute to the situation?"

"Have I felt this way before?"

"What happened before when I was feeling this?"

"What do I want to have happen instead?"

"Is this a pattern?"

"What beliefs are operating here?"

"Un-glomph" your emotions. One thing people do that intensifies their emotions is to take one piece of evidence and generalize it to all of life. One slip-up means they're a failure. For instance, I used to think I was dumb in general. My evidence was that I didn't do well in math. That's what I now call "glomphing" things up.

So beware when the thoughts accompanying your emotions include "always" or "never." Investigate the specifics. For example, if you're judging yourself as inadequate, ask yourself when you feel that way and when you don't. Do you feel inadequate only about your weight? Do you feel inadequate socially? Financially? Why? Are you unfairly comparing yourself to others? Are you setting unrealistic goals? Do you ignore your strengths?

You might find out you're not as inadequate as you originally thought. Even if you find you still feel inadequate in a particular area, you don't have to view yourself as defective in general. Just decide whether it's worth it for you to learn more in this area. For instance, I'm inadequate at fixing cars, but that's okay with me because I'm not really interested in fixing cars, and I'm very good at other things. The point is, try to be fair in your self-assessments.

Recognize and change your negative tapes. Here's an example of what I mean. One of my students complained that she felt nervous and insecure at a party. When we looked at what she was thinking, she realized that before she even arrived at the party, she was making pictures in her head of herself behaving and speaking awkwardly, and people rejecting her as a result. She was responding to these images rather than to the actual people, who were actually friendly. So whenever she caught herself running those negative tapes, she recalled times when she felt confident and secure.

Seek help. You might find it necessary to consult a therapist to help you figure out what's really going on with your feelings. Many of us have trouble seeing clearly through our emotions because we don't want to know what's "wrong" with us, and we're caught up in our misconceptions. Even therapists, including myself, get consultations when we want to resolve an issue or move ourselves to peak performance in some area.

How to Keep Your Cool As Your Pounds Melt Away

Losing weight is no piece of cake. Dieting can leave you emotionally tense and physically irritable. But it doesn't have to be torture, either. Here are some tips to counteract the feelings of resentment and deprivation that sometimes make dieting an agony for body and soul alike. The advice is courtesy of Michael R. Lowe, Ph.D., associate professor in the Clinical Psychology Division at Hahnemann University Hospital in Philadelphia.

Ask yourself if you really need to lose weight. "Many people who are dissatisfied with their size aren't really overweight, but they're either on a diet or feel they should be," says Dr. Lowe. If you have good reason to feel fat, though—if you weigh 20 percent or more above the recommended weight for your height and/or you have weight-related health problems—then you may need to face some facts.

Accept the challenge to change. Get used to the fact that you will never be able to eat whatever you like, whenever you like, in any amount, without gaining weight. "If people want to lose weight and keep it off, they first have to accept the fact that they will never be able to return to their eating habits of the past," says Dr. Lowe. "In our program, we find it useful to describe an overweight tendency as a kind of handicap. And as with other physical handicaps, the people who ultimately adapt best are those who can get past the feelings of anger and injustice, strive toward new goals, and develop new feelings of pride at having overcome their 'handicap.' "

Don't cut back drastically. "Drastic efforts—a few weeks of strict discipline and extreme self-sacrifice—are usually followed by a return to old eating habits, leaving people feeling guilty and disgusted with themselves," says Dr. Lowe. "Instead, cut back gradually."

Don't adopt very odd or specialized diets. "Highly idiosyncratic diets that force you to eat only a few foods will also leave you feeling very deprived," says Dr. Lowe. You're apt to feel edgy and irritable. Odd diets are also hard to follow if you work outside the home, attend social functions, or otherwise lead a normal, active life.

Build indulgences into your program. "If you say, 'I'm never going to eat ice cream again for the rest of my life,' you are aiming for the impossible and setting yourself up for failure," says Dr. Lowe. "Black-or-white, all-or-nothing thinking can undermine the very thing you're trying to achieve. So allow yourself an occasional stop for an ice cream cone (but don't keep a half-gallon carton in the freezer)."

Congratulate yourself on the victories and a healthier way of life. "If you lock yourself in a mind-set of 'How much longer can I endure this?' you will feel upset, frustrated and angry," says Dr. Lowe. "But if you focus on the healthful benefits of weight control, feelings of inferiority and deprivation give way to pride, and your new diet becomes a morale booster."

Plan ahead. It's one thing to be obsessed with food (which many dieters are) and quite another to plan ahead in order to stick to your diet.

"Weight-conscious people need to be more mindful of what they're going to eat and not make on-the-spot decisions at mealtime," says Dr. Lowe. Otherwise, you may end up eating high-calorie foods by default.

"Plan menus, shop for food, prepare for food-centered

situations," says Dr. Lowe. "If you're going to a party, prepare to decline food when it's offered. Or set limits to how
much you will eat. Or eat sparingly earlier that day."

Don't let others coax or bully you off your diet.
"No one, hosts and hostesses included, has the right to
pressure you into eating or drinking something you
shouldn't," says Dr. Lowe.

Losing weight is no piece of cake. But it doesn't have
to be torture, either.

Dealing with the Critics

Like many overweight people, you may be self-conscious about your weight. You'd like to lose, but until you
do, you have to deal with comments about your weight,
including those from well-meaning friends who, thanks to
a great metabolism, have never weighed more than
110 pounds in their life. Or those who say "so and so is
on a diet and you could really lose weight, too—you're
way too heavy, you know." Or going to a doctor's office for
any reason and having the staff and/or doctor shake their
head or act as if the number on the scale is indicative of
some kind of moral failure.

What can you do?

Your experience is all too common in this society.
"The harassment and ridicule fat people are faced with on
a daily basis prevents many of us from leaving our homes
except for the most compelling reasons," says Sally Smith,
executive director of the National Association to Advance
Fat Acceptance (NAAFA). "Will the average fat person go
to a public pool, where she will be called a beached
whale? Will the average fat person confront the owner of
a car with a bumper sticker that says, 'Save the Whales,
Harpoon a Fat Chick'? Will the average fat person walk
down the street eating an ice cream cone? No way! One
woman I know was doing just that, and a stranger came

up to her, grabbed the ice cream cone out of her hand, threw it to the ground, and said it should be a crime for her to be eating an ice cream cone. Strangers have called me 'disgusting,' even when I'm dressed professionally."

It's no wonder you might feel crushed if you've endured years of such insensitive remarks. But you can learn to feel less hurt by such comments. People's remarks can't force you to feel bad. It's the view you take of them that can make you feel bad. You can learn to think and respond differently so that you can retain your sense of self-worth even in the face of disapproval. Remember—the comments are a reflection on the person who says them, not a reflection on your worth.

Stand Up for Yourself

Smith has a few ideas on how to deal with snide remarks from strangers. "Once a group of businessmen were making fat jokes about one of my friends," says Smith. "She went up to one of them and said, 'If you had your wish, would you rather be fat or stupid?' He said, 'I'd rather be stupid.' And she said, 'Well, you got your wish.'

"Sometimes I say, 'I can't believe there are so many fat bigots in the world' or 'I wonder if they make ethnic jokes, too.' Other times, I'll go up to them and say, 'I think that you probably don't understand much what it's like to be fat in this society. Let me tell you what a typical day in my life is like.' I'll educate them, and say, 'Regardless of my weight, I shouldn't have to put up with this.'

"As for your doctor, you can say, 'I'm not here because of my weight. I'm here for my flu,' " recommends Smith. "You can refuse to be weighed—there's usually no compelling medical reason you need to be weighed. I tell nurses I don't do scales anymore."

If you still feel your doctor is insensitive, you need to find a better doctor. Before you go to a new doctor, you can interview the doctor or his or her staff and ask how they feel about fat people and whether they make weight an issue if it's unrelated to the condition. Often, local NAAFA chapters have word-of-mouth referrals for fat-friendly doctors.

Be Assertive

To deal with well-meaning friends and family, Judi Hollis, Ph.D., founder and clinical director of Helping Overeaters thru People and Education, recommends the following assertive techniques.

Agree with the truthful part. For example, if a relative tells you, "You are fat and ugly," you could reply, "I am big, aren't I?" If you don't necessarily agree, you can just admit the possibility the other person is correct. For instance, if someone says, "You're going to die if you keep eating like that," you could simply say, "You may be right."

Why? Denying often encourages an argument. This method, on the other hand, helps you acknowledge your weight or eating behaviors without thinking that you're "wrong." In effect, you're saying, "It may be true. But so what?"

Ask questions. You can ask people to be more specific about how they feel. For instance, if a friend tells you to lose weight, you can ask, "Why do you think I *haven't* been trying to lose weight? Explain to me why you are disappointed." Or ask, "How does this affect you?" This way, you can understand your friend's opinions and feelings without having to accept them as your own.

Express your feelings. Your well-meaning friends probably don't realize that their comments sting you. Letting them know how you feel without accusing them of bad intentions may help her change her ways. For instance, you could say:

"I'm hurt by your criticism."

"I'm afraid you don't like me."

"I feel bad about disappointing you."

"I'm embarrassed by my fat."

"I feel a lot of pressure when you ask about my weight."

Make a request. For instance, you might say, "I really need you to accept me the way I am and stop commenting about my weight."

Compliments: Learn to Love 'Em!
By Marilee Goldberg, Ph.D.

People who are overweight yearn for compliments, whether they're 1 pound or 100 pounds heavy.

Ironically, many of us are so used to negative feedback that we can't even acknowledge the compliments when they do come. Deep down inside, we believe we don't really deserve such praise. Someone once complimented me on how nice I looked, and instead of saying thank you, I told her I'd gotten my dress on sale.

Many people actually need to be trained in the art of giving and receiving compliments. The reward? They gradually move from self-conscious and shy to self-confident and smiling. And since the ability to give and receive compliments and support is so important in creating intimacy, another wonderful consequence is that people begin to deepen and enrich their relationships with the important others in their lives.

But learning to accept compliments does more than help you grow personally. It's an essential part of managing your weight. After all, most of us are really hungry for affection, not food.

What Is a Compliment?

A real compliment is sincere and honest. It can come in the form of words or gestures, like a pat on the back. You can receive a compliment from someone else or give it to yourself. A compliment simply lets another person know that you admire something about them.

There are essentially two kinds of compliments. The first kind is about something a person has done: "Congratulations on a job well done." The other is less obvious, praising a person for their way of being: "Thanks for being so tactful and supportive," or "I really appreciate your warmth and humor." Both kinds are important.

Become a Compliment Detective

So how are you doing with compliments in your own life? The only way to find out is to start paying attention. Listen to how people in your family speak with each other. Are they encouraging of each other or not? Listen for compliments. Do you hear any? If yes, listen for what kind they are, how they are delivered, and how they are received. If there are few compliments, listen for opportunities to begin giving them.

Do the same thing in your job and with your friends. Begin to listen to the "compliment customs" of the people in your life and figure out whether you're happy with the way it is or if there could be more "goodies" for everybody. You may even want to "interview" people and find out from them how they think and feel about giving and receiving compliments.

The Art of Giving

The next thing you can do is give a few compliments to others and observe how easy or difficult it is for you. Do you feel comfortable and natural? Give yourself a pat on the back if you do. If not, start practicing in small, easy steps. In general, it is much easier to give the "doing" kind of compliment than the "being" kind. So tell someone that you think they did a good job, or that the color of their sweater is perfect for them. When you have some experience with this kind of compliment, you can risk the more intimate "being" compliments, like "I get so much pleasure out of being with you."

Another part of being a skillful "giver" involves learning what a person is most proud of or cares about most. It's more effective to tell your best friend that you love the living room remodeling she just did than to compliment the hairstyle she's been wearing for years.

The Art of Receiving

Now, here's the really hard part: What happens when someone gives you a compliment? Can you accept the compliment gracefully and simply say thank you? Does your body stay relaxed, or do you get a bit uncomfortable? If you're like so many others, you may actually tense up a bit or get flushed if it's difficult for you to be on the receiving end. But remember that a compliment is really a spoken gift. If someone gave you a beautifully wrapped present, you probably wouldn't give it back and say, "Sorry, I can't accept this." Yet that's exactly what happens when someone says, "You look great," and you answer, "Oh, that's not true. I just gained weight."

One useful exercise is called "The Beauty I See in You." Each person in a group or class gets to stand in the center and be "it." Everyone else takes turns telling that person about something they appreciate in them. Participants are often embarrassed at the beginning, but by the time they've done this exercise several times, they really enjoy being on both the giving and receiving end.

Complimenting Ourselves

Giving yourself a compliment is simply a version of positive self-talk, and it's a great habit to cultivate! If you practice enough, those positive thoughts will become an automatic part of your everyday talks with yourself.

Have you ever noticed that, in life, people usually find what they're looking for? If you're looking for beauty in yourself and the people around you, you'll usually find it. If you're looking for faults...well, they're all too easy to find.

If you look for the positive in people, they'll want to be around you more. And they'll be happier when they are around you. Now that sounds to me like a pretty rewarding way to live. And it's just a matter of practice.

Are You Bulimic?
Ask Yourself These Questions

Eating disorders have attracted huge public interest. But few people understand just what eating disorders are. The term "bulimic," for example, is commonly understood as someone who deliberately vomits after eating. And that's a big misconception.

Not every bulimic forces vomiting. And not everyone who vomits after eating is considered to be bulimic. Here's the official medical definition that psychiatrists use in diagnosing bulimia.

• Recurrent episodes of binge eating (rapid consumption of a large amount of food in a short period of time, usually less than 2 hours)
• At least three of the following: consumption of easily ingested, high-calorie food during a binge; inconspicuous eating during a binge; termination of eating episodes by abdominal pain, sleep, social interruption, or self-induced vomiting; repeated attempts to lose weight by severely restrictive diets, self-induced vomiting, or use of cathartics or diuretics; frequent weight fluctuations of greater than 10 pounds due to alternating binges and fasts

• Awareness that the eating pattern is abnormal and fear of not being able to stop eating voluntarily
• Depressed mood and self-deprecating thoughts following eating binges

If you have some or all of these symptoms, write to the American Anorexia-Bulimia Association, 418 East 76th Street, New York, NY 10021. The association can send information and refer you to a clinic, therapist, or self-help group in your area. Or call your state psychological association, which can refer you to a psychologist who specializes in eating disorders.

Attitude Adjustments That Banish Binges

What makes some people go on voracious binges, then feel depressed and guilty?

Irrational beliefs are at the root of it all, psychologists Barbara G. Bauer, Ph.D., and Wayne P. Anderson, Ph.D., reported in the *Journal of Counseling and Development*. Based on their experience with bulimic clients, they identified nine common beliefs that perpetuate eating disorders and described how to debunk them. Even if you don't have full-blown bulimia, you might find that this advice may help diminish your eating or weight problems.

Dr. Bauer gave special permission to report her findings and her recommendations. The following beliefs are presented in what is thought to be the order of frequency, with the most frequent appearing first.

1. Being or becoming overweight is the worst thing that can happen to me. Fat is disgusting and repulsive. To be fat is to be a failure. "This belief is probably the most universal belief held by individuals with eating disorders," explain Dr. Bauer and Dr. Anderson, who are coauthors of the book *Bulimia: Book for Therapist and Client.* "Many have been [or are] obese as adolescents and have painful memories of teasing and rejection because of their weight. Even more than the average woman, these women accept the societal standard equating slenderness with attractiveness."

Women with bulimia believe they're fat and disgusting even though they really are at a healthy weight. The constant self-deprecation for obesity, whether it's real or imagined, is a major contributor to continued binge eating and depression, says Dr. Bauer.

"Disputing this belief with the opinion that 'You look fine' has little effect," say the psychologists. "Part of the problem is that society, to some extent, supports this belief."

The solution? They recommend the technique of thought stopping. Whenever self-criticizing thoughts begin, say *"stop!"* loudly to yourself. Then turn your thoughts to a neutral topic until you can return to kinder thoughts.

2. Certain foods are good foods; others are bad foods. "Diet" foods are good foods. Fattening foods are bad. Eating bad foods makes me a bad person; eating good foods makes makes me a good person. Bad food is turned directly into body fat. The first foods declared to be "bad" are usually fats and sweets, such as chocolate, butter, desserts, and such. The next foods to be banished are often the complex carbohydrates such as pasta, potatoes, and breads, even though these foods really aren't fattening.

One problem with these beliefs is that after eating only "good" low-calorie foods, you may feel so deprived and hungry that you binge on "bad" foods. And the guilt resulting from being "bad" just makes you feel worse and may prompt you to eat even more to make you feel better. So these strict rules don't even keep you away from the foods you're trying to avoid!

"Good and bad foods do not exist," assert Dr. Bauer and Dr. Anderson. "It is diets lacking selections from all food groups that can create deficiencies."

They advise gradually trying foods on your bad food list. It may help reduce anxiety if you talk to yourself calmly or relax yourself before you eat. It may also be helpful to reframe the eating of forbidden foods as taking "medicine" to prevent binge eating.

And remember—small amounts of forbidden food *won't* turn directly into large amounts of body fat. "Four ounces of chocolate is only a quarter of a pound," point out the authors. "Even if you absorbed 100 percent of it, which is unlikely, it would still be only a quarter of a pound. Not even you can disobey the laws of physics and create matter from nothing."

3. I must have control over all my actions to feel safe. Minor dietary indiscretions are indicative of a complete loss of self-control. Trying harder is the answer to my food problems. "Many clients attempt to regain control of their food behavior after a binge/purge episode by severely restricting food intake," say Dr. Bauer and Dr. Anderson. "This results in intense hunger, which often perpetuates the binge/purge/restrict cycle. It is often helpful to recommend eating a small meal after purging. This recommendation is initially responded to with dismay; however, if the client will eat and retain a small meal after purging, the cycle of recurrent binge eating prompted by hunger can be broken. We usually recommend a meal that is a mixture of protein and carbohydrate, such as cheese and crackers or yogurt. These are frequently 'safe foods' and not likely to prompt a purge. It is not uncommon for women to cut down their binge/purge episodes by 50 percent with this technique."

4. I must do everything perfectly or what I do is worthless. I hold myself to standards that I would never apply to another individual. I feel that, regardless of performance, I could have done even better

if I had tried harder. People who hold these beliefs often have trouble accepting compliments. They are quick to point out flaws in their performance and discount the accomplishment.

If this sounds familiar, you could tell a close friend or spouse about this tendency and request them to confront you if you try to negate a compliment. If you accomplish something and don't acknowledge it, your friend could say, "You must be pleased with the way you did that."

Another way to tackle your feeling of failure is to make a list of at least two things you felt good about doing each day before you go to sleep.

And to attack the rigidity involved in perfectionism, Dr. Bauer and Dr. Anderson prescribe imperfection. "We instruct our clients to begin at least two things each day and deliberately leave them unfinished," say the psychologists. "Some examples are to leave one corner of your bed unmade; start a letter but quit in the middle of a sentence; balance half of your checkbook. Clients are amused by the assignment at first but soon find out how unsettling it is. Considerable insight is often gained into how rigid their need to be perfect has made them."

5. Everyone is aware of and interested in what I am doing. If I hear people laughing, I know it is about me. Other people watch and are critical of what I eat and know if I have gained weight. Here's a way to challenge your belief that others can notice small changes in you: Try regularly weighing yourself without looking at the number and have someone else check it for you. Then guess if there has been a gain or a loss and if so, how much. Dr. Bauer says that when her clients find out how inaccurate their own estimates are, they quickly realize that others couldn't possibly notice small changes.

And if you're self-conscious while eating with others, try eating with a trusted friend or therapist alone. When you're comfortable with this, try eating with the friend in a small restaurant. You'll probably discover that nothing terrible happens.

6. Everyone must love me and approve of what I do. I perceive rejection whether it is intended or not. I feel unworthy of love. If you have these beliefs, you may take even minor corrections as evidence of failure and rejection. You may find reasons to reject people before they can reject you.

The main way to realize you're acceptable no matter what is to experience consistent acceptance from a counselor or a close, trusted friend, says Dr. Bauer. As you reveal your innermost secrets, the ones that make you believe that they're bad, and the counselor responds in an empathetic manner, the intensity of your belief starts to fade.

Many people with this belief have friendships and family relationships that are based on their being a caregiver, because they believe you're so unworthy of love they have to earn it. "As the client begins to recognize the one-sided nature of these relationships, she may attempt to elicit support from these individuals," say Dr. Bauer and Dr. Anderson. "It may be necessary to encourage the client to expand her circle of friends. One of the best settings for this is in group therapy, where mutual support is encouraged. It may take a while for the client to become comfortable with allowing others to give to her, but the results are often closer friendships than ever experienced before."

7. External validation is everything. Numbers are very important: calories, weight, grade point average, score on any type of competition. I take opinion polls every time I need to make a decision to be sure I am making the right choice. "With some of our clients, numbers become a way of competing with oneself," say Dr. Bauer and Dr. Anderson. "Each time a new level of success is reached, nothing less is acceptable. For example, if the client usually jogs 2 miles per day but manages to push herself to 2½ miles one day, 2 miles is never good enough again."

This kind of striving often comes from the belief that you're valued for what you do, not for who you are. So recognize the superficial nature of measurements and focus on unconditional self-acceptance.

Dr. Bauer encourages her clients to try new activities even though they may not be the best at them. You'll know you're getting rid of this niggling belief if you can be comfortable saying, "I did the best I could, and that's good enough."

8. As soon as *[a particular event]* occurs, I will be able to give up bulimia. Some of the popular events thought to end binge eating for good include graduating from school, getting a job, leaving home, getting married, and getting pregnant. Sometimes this so-called magical thinking is connected to weight loss: "If I could only lose 5 more pounds, then I could quit." If the anticipated event should happen and the bulimia continues, another event is quickly substituted.

"The most effective force in disputing the irrational beliefs is interaction in group therapy," say the psychologists. "Other group members are quick to point out the denial involved in magical thinking. There frequently is a confrontation from a group member who has accomplished whatever goal the individual has set up and is still struggling with the eating disorder."

9. To be successful, a woman must combine the traditional values of women with the aggressive career orientation of men. I must be dependent and subservient like my mother; aggressive and competitive like my father; and feminine but never sexual. "Since these expectations are of opposing positions, no matter what the person does, she feels she is disappointing someone," says Dr. Bauer. "But as she goes through therapy and begins to formulate her own life goals and definition of her role as a woman, she often finds that the expected disapproval from her parents does not happen. Much of what she anticipated happening when she 'disappoints' her parents exists in her own mind. If the parents do try to control her, the counselor can rehearse some defensive listening techniques to help the client deflect their efforts."

The counselor and patient must have an understanding of what these nine beliefs are, if change in behavior is to occur.

Keeping It Light:
How to Add Laughter to Weight Loss

There's no doubt about it—trying to lose weight is usually no fun at all. Recently, though, weight-loss experts have begun introducing ways to help you turn the pain to laughter by bringing humor into the process.

Take the approach of registered dietitian Robin Flipse. She helped her weight-loss class get through the torture of weigh-ins by using a cartoon. The drawing showed a large woman stepping onto a scale. Everybody wrote a caption to express their own rationalizations, hopes and fears. Here are some examples:

"If only I were 11 inches taller."

"I had no idea this dress was this heavy."

"Oh, please, scale, say that I'm down to 110, so I'll look really good and I'll meet someone, and we'll fall in love and get married and I'll be happy for the rest of my life."

Another cartoon she used with a cardiac rehabilitation class shows a middle-aged man jogging in a park. Pinned to the back of his sweat suit is a sign that says, "I'd rather be smoking, drinking, and eating."

"I use cartoons because it's fun, and people are more

receptive to learning when they're having a good time," explains Flipse, who conducted the presentation "Cartoons as a Method of Nutrition Education" at an American Dietetic Association (ADA) meeting. "It also conveys sympathy and understanding for the thoughts and feelings you may have about weight loss. After all, many people would rather not exercise or cut fat. In a group setting, cartoons and other methods of humor help to reduce the feeling of being alone. They are all laughing at one thing, that is, the cartoon with the chains around the refrigerator. It gives the group a sense of bonding because they all share in the same battle."

But Flipse warns, "Humor cannot be too clownish. The instructor must be careful in the selection and presentation of the cartoons. If abused, participants will lose respect for the instructor and thus lose the benefit of that class."

Flipse finds "Cathy" cartoons a great source of humor and inspiration. "There was a cartoon where Cathy was coming home from a date, and her mother says, 'Well, how did your date go?' and Cathy's carrying a gigantic container of rum raisin ice cream in one hand and a gigantic container of mocha almond in the other," says Flipse. "Of course, the implied answer is, 'The date was lousy; I'm going to eat my troubles away.' I use that cartoon when I make the point that your weight is vulnerable as long as you turn to food for emotional relief."

Looking at your problems through the eyes of humor can help you confront your problems with less pain. "In order to laugh at yourself, you have to forgive yourself for not being perfect," says Mark Therrien, who also promoted humor at the ADA conference and who directs InnerPlay, an organization that promotes the therapeutic use of humor and play. "And the forgiving attitude allows you to look at your mistakes, learn from them...and laugh at them. Besides, laughing burns calories."

Here are some ways to "lighten up" your weight-loss program.

• If you're looking for a dietitian or some other counselor to help you lose weight, find someone who has a sense of humor you can appreciate. "Usually learning is equated with hard work, but you'll learn more about nutrition and weight loss if you're having fun," points out Flipse.
• Collect cartoons with which you can identify. It should be easy—many of the daily funnies are about eating and weight.
• Create your own cartoons with your own drawings, or with pictures cut out of magazines and your own captions.

CHAPTER

5

THE 92 BEST
TIPS OF 1992

The hardest part of losing weight is getting through those times when you most want to "pig out" and you least want to work out. Motivation dwindles. Dieting just seems too hard. At times like these you need all the help you can get to stay on track. This chapter gives you the top weight-loss strategies for 1992, compiled from the pages of diet, food, and exercise books, and interviews with the experts. You'll find super-fast tips on everything from cooking leaner to harnessing your hunger to burning more calories with your exercise! Read them all and give some of them a try. You'll find the way to weight loss just got easier.

13 Illuminating Tips for Nighttime Snackers

1. Set a deadline. Decide on a time after which you do not eat (e.g., no food after 7 P.M.).

2. Drink plenty of water. This will quench your thirst and give you a sense of fullness.

3. Reduce television watching. Watching the TV goes hand in hand with snacking, especially late at night. You can also try to substitute noneating activities for snacking during television viewing (e.g., riding a stationary bike or knitting).

4. Exercise in the evening. It will help reduce your appetite.

5. Go for a brisk walk after dinner. Take the kids or the dog for a refreshing stroll.

6. Get out of the kitchen. You might even want to leave the house for a little while after dinner.

7. Do your food shopping after a meal. If you shop when you're hungry, everything edible seems much more tempting.

8. Make a well-balanced breakfast a morning ritual. Realizing that breakfast is only a few hours away may help you stave off the midnight munchies.

9. Avoid skimpy lunches. Eat a well-balanced noontime meal.

10. Avoid meal skipping, self-starvation, and low-calorie dieting. These noneating behaviors inevitably trigger binge eating at vulnerable times (like at bedtime).

11. Limit your snacking. Snack only during daytime hours if eating in the evening seems to trigger binges.

12. Establish a regular routine. Pick a time for eating and a time for exercise. Then stick to them. (Be patient with yourself; old habits die hard!)

13. Join a health club. Work out in the evenings. On nonworkout nights enjoy a sauna or massage.

Cooking Right

14. Microwave to zap more fat. Microwaving eliminates the fat from ground beef better than any other cooking method, nutritionists say. And a test with today's new extra-low-fat ground beef confirmed that distinction. Superlean ground beef (5 to 10 percent fat) retained less fat when it was microwaved on paper towels than when it was roasted, broiled, or pan-fried in an electric skillet in a laboratory at Texas A&M University.

◆

15. Cook with nonstick pots and pans. You won't have to add as much oil. Or use a nonstick, nonfat cooking spray such as Pam.

16. Watch where you wok. Chinese cookbooks may tell you to use 3 or 4 tablespoons of oil in the wok. Too much, says David Keh of David K's, a restaurant in New York. He uses no more than 2 teaspoons for four servings.

17. Change your oil. Fancy New York restaurants are serving baked potatoes with a splash of olive oil instead of butter or sour cream. Pasta salad made with olive oil and wine vinegar instead of mayonnaise derives half as many of its calories from fat.

18. Go easy on the eggs. Make your omelets with three egg whites but only two yolks, or mix whole eggs half-and-half with Egg Beaters or another egg substitute.

19. Prop up your poultry. A vertical poultry roaster keeps a bird upright so the fat can drip away as it cooks. The meat stays moist and cooks evenly without basting with butter or oil. Bonus: Poultry cooks faster.

20. Deemphasize the meat. Make stews and stir-fries that use meat as a condiment or seasoning instead of as the mainstay of a meal.

21. Sneak in the turkey. Replace ground beef in chili, lasagna, meat loaf, spaghetti sauce, and casseroles with ground turkey or chicken breast. And while hamburgers made entirely of ground turkey tend to be more than a bit on the dry side, a little ground turkey mixed with ground beef is hardly noticeable.

22. Take a word from the peanut gallery. Most major brands of peanut butter are made with hydrogenated (saturated) vegetable oil. Try fresh-ground peanut butter instead. Find it at the supermarket or health-food store.

23. Try a new take on steak. Rather than buying fatty cuts like New York strip or Delmonico, try flank steak, which is leaner. Broil it and be sure to slice it across the grain. You'll get a tender meat with a lot less fat.

24. Marinate from 8 'til 8. Marinating a piece of raw meat in the refrigerator overnight can make it more tender and give it a better flavor, so you may not miss the fat you trimmed off. A can of tomato soup, beef broth, or onion soup makes a easy marinade, or use a mixture of ¼ cup of red wine vinegar, some minced garlic, and a tablespoon of Worcestershire sauce.

25. Don't be fooled by imitations. In case you don't read labels, fake mozzarella cheese has 90 calories and 7 grams of fat per ounce, while real mozzarella cheese has 80 calories and 5 grams of fat. To make matters worse, the imitation stuff has less protein and more sodium. True, it has no cholesterol—but real mozzarella has only 10 milligrams per ounce.

26. Get to know your cows. Limousin cattle, a French breed, arrived in America about 20 years ago. Some cuts are better than 95 percent fat free, and the top sirloin has nearly 46 percent less fat than other choice sirloins tested.

Golden Trim, another brand of low-fat beef, is between 91 and 98 percent fat free. It's available in supermarkets in the Northeast, Southwest, and West, so far. Two cuts, the beef tip rounds and top round, are lower in total fat than the same amount of skinless chicken.

27. Learn a new language. Certain foreign cooking terms actually translate to "fat added." Sauté means "add

butter." Tempura means "fried in batter." Au gratin indicates the dish has cheese sauce. Broiling sounds safe, and
it is—unless it's in butter.

28. Favor fish. Almost any way you measure it, fish
has less fat than beef or poultry. Flounder, for instance,
contains only about half the fat of chicken. Spare your fish
the deep fryer, though. Fried fish fillets are about 65 percent fat; the same fish when baked contains less than half
that much fat.

29. Try shellfish. Although lobster and shrimp are
rather high in cholesterol, they're low in saturated fat.
Clams and scallops contain less than half the fat of roast
chicken without skin. Eat them steamed or broiled rather
than fried or stuffed.

30. And try shelf-fish. Look for canned tuna packed
in water; you don't need the added vegetable oil. Tuna in
water is moist enough for making sandwiches, especially
when you add lettuce and tomato and a bit of low-fat
mayonnaise.

31. Miss the mayo. The main ingredient in tartar
sauce is mayonnaise. If you can't marinate fish, try broiling
it in a little lemon juice with some herbs and spices sprin-
kled on both sides.

32. Make 'waves. Instead of cooking fish and vegetables in butter, reduce the fat by microwaving them using
lemon and herbs.

33. Use the right stuffing. Poultry stuffings made of
bread ingredients absorb fat drippings from the bird. Go
light on the bread and heavy on sliced citrus fruit and
spices.

34. Join the gold rush. Look for a variety of potatoes going by the names of Yukon Gold, Yellow Finnish, or Yellow Rose. Most potatoes you see are white types, which lack the flavor that these golden ones have. Whether you bake them, microwave them, roast them, steam them, or grill them, they cook up with a moist, buttery flavor, which means you don't have to add as much butter.

35. Drink, but think. The *occasional* use of liquid diet drinks (particularly to avoid skipping breakfast or lunch) can help give your diet a boost, even if you only have a few pounds to lose. Make sure the product contains about a third of the recommended daily allowances of vitamins and minerals (the label will tell). Use the shakes for only one or two meals a day—ideally for breakfast or lunch—and eat a low-fat dinner.

Eating Light

36. Eat slowly. If you're a fast eater, you may be finishing your plate long before your stomach has had a chance to send the signal that it's satisfied. Slow down and you'll eat less. Another reason: Food eaten in a rush may be more readily stored as fat.

37. Orchestrate your meals. Studies suggest that people eat more slowly when they listen to soft, slow music. In contrast, Maria Simonson, Ph.D., Sc.D., director of the Health, Weight, and Stress Program at Johns Hopkins Medical Institutions in Baltimore, says, "rock-and-rollers practically inhale food."

38. Paint the kitchen. Calm, soothing colors slow your eating. Warm, sensuous colors make you pig out. Consider painting your dining area a cool blue and serving

◆

your meals on dark-brown, blue, dull gray, or plain white plates.

39. Put pencil to paper. A Weight Watchers study of 26 people who had lost at least 40 pounds and kept it off for a year found that 95 percent of them followed a written dieting plan. This is, of course, the Weight Watchers philosophy. Yes, it works.

40. Start your day right. Eat breakfast, and make it high-fiber. Cereals containing high fiber contain the fewest calories per serving and tend to quell your appetite longest.

41. Enjoy what you eat. "You don't have to eat sawdust to lose weight," says Mark Friedman, Ph.D., assistant director of the Monell Chemical Senses Center in Philadelphia. "A palatable diet is not going to make you overeat. If you eat lower-calorie foods that taste good, at least you won't have to worry about giving up the good taste." Suggestions: meats like lean sirloin (trim the fat), turkey, and chicken; vegetables like potatoes, green beans, and broccoli; fruits like oranges, apples, and honeydew melon; seafood like lobster (hold the butter), salmon, and flounder.

42. Choose an angel over a devil. Some folks with a sweet tooth crave candy, while others take the cake. If you go window-shopping at bakeries, consider angel food sponge. It's low in calories and made with almost no fat.

43. Lighten your lightener. Lighten your coffee— and soups and sauces, for that matter—with evaporated skim milk instead of half-and-half or whole milk. You'll still get rich body, but with very little fat.

44. Give your bagel the slip. Neufchâtel cheese contains somewhat less fat and fewer calories than cream cheese, and is similar in texture and taste. You'll find Neufchâtel at most supermarkets.

45. Change the way you say "cheese." Skim-milk cheeses contain the least fat of any type of cheese, but you may be put off by their somewhat bland flavor. Try them melted in grilled cheese sandwiches. For cold sandwiches or snacking, use part-skim-milk cheeses. Lifetime makes some that taste fairly close to whole-milk cheeses but contain one-half to two-thirds less fat and cholesterol. They're available at supermarkets and health-food stores.

46. Choose nonalcoholic booze. Some alcoholic beverages deliver more calories than rich desserts. When you're having more than one drink, make the second one sparkling water or a nonalcoholic beer. "Alcohol is a sneak," says Nancy Cohen, Ph.D., registered dietitian and assistant professor of nutrition at the University of Massachusetts. "Every gram of alcohol is 7 calories, whether you're drinking beer or wine."

47. Try a toasted treat. For a low-fat snack, top French bread or pita wedges with grated Parmesan, low-fat ricotta, or low-fat cottage cheese. Sprinkle on pepper or herbs, and toast.

48. Got a cold? Put your diet on hold! "Minor illnesses may require a modest increase in foods rich in vitamins and minerals and a total diet adequate in protein and calories," says dietitian Ann Coulston of Stanford University. "There's a good chance you'll feel better faster if you make sure you're meeting your calorie and nutrient needs in a properly balanced diet." And don't forget plenty of fluids.

49. Mind your mayo. Hidden in every cup of regular mayonnaise is one egg yolk, which contains not only cho-

◆

lesterol but a considerable amount of saturated fat. Most mayonnaise makers now sell versions that are lower in calories and cholesterol. They're not bad.

50. Don't get dark. Chocolate contains lots of saturated fat. The darker and more bitter the bar, the more fat it contains. Milk chocolate gets about 30 percent of its calories from fat; bittersweet, about 45 percent. So when you have to have it, know what's in it.

51. Go cold chicken. Hillshire Farm makes well-seasoned, low-fat luncheon meats called Deli Select. The smoked chicken breast is 98 percent fat-free and weighs in at only 10 calories per slice.

52. Eat less often. You're probably not really hungry for those food-filled coffee breaks. You can enjoy the company of friends over a cup of coffee or sugar-free soft drink.

53. Serve it up smaller. Learn to be content with one serving. One cookie tastes just like a handful. Put less food on the table. Serve smaller desserts by cutting a pie into eight or ten pieces.

54. Keep temptation out of sight. Clear away food immediately after meals and put snack foods away. Can you get along without those dishes of candy and nuts?

Maintain Your Motivation

55. Do it for yourself. A very common reason for wanting to lose weight is to look good for someone else. Shedding pounds for partners "is a sure prescription for failure," says Robert E. T. Stark, M.D., chairman of the board of the American Society of Bariatric Physicians. "If you are dieting for any reason that is not internally motivated, you are unlikely to succeed."

56. Be positive. Wanting to lose weight for reasons such as hating how you look or wanting to be more successful at work—good reasons though they are—is not a great motivator. Instead, think of what you'll gain: self-esteem, energy, health, sexual vitality.

57. Be reasonable! Diets can be beastly embroilments of unreasonable (and often unhealthy) goals, leavened with frustration, guilt, and recrimination. Since strict dieting can put the brakes on long-term weight control, you'll actually do better if you take it easy.

58. It's *not* all or nothing. Many people quit their diets when they suffer a temporary dietary setback: One little chocolate bar—or even an entire day of eating everything within reach—is no reason to give up. That's an example of all-or-nothing thinking, and it is completely unrealistic. "People have to realize that the process of weight loss is uneven," Cohen says. "People do slip up, and that's okay. If the end goal is life change, then it's going to take some time to get used to."

59. Weigh-ins are way out! When you're looking for immediate gratification, you may be inclined to step on the scale every day to monitor your progress. But if you're losing weight correctly, you shouldn't be losing a lot every day. A few ounces isn't going to look like much on that scale. Don't lose heart, just *stop weighing yourself.* A better measure of progress, according to Frederick C. Hagerman, Ph.D., an exercise physiologist at Ohio University, is simply this: After you've been working at it a while, you should be able to pull your belt back a notch.

60. Be sure you're ready. So you say you're going to get a new job, spend more time with the kids, improve your sex life and, oh, yes, lose that spare tire. Resolution overload is pretty common. If dieting is low on your list, do yourself a favor and hold off until you have a realistic chance of success.

Mind over Platter

61. Visualize your thinner thighs. Visualization is a powerful tool for building willpower, Dr. Simonson says. For example, if you want to lose weight for better health, imagine playing ball with a grandchild when you're 70. If you want to gain energy and strength, envision an activity, such as backpacking, that requires those qualities.

62. Don't go on a diet. "Diet" implies a short-term commitment. Calorie-restrictive diets don't work in the long run. Most popular diets put a cap of 1,000 calories on daily food allowed. That's not enough sustenance and can lead to nutrient deficiencies. "What usually happens on these diets is that within a week to ten days people complain of having symptoms of the flu, even though they don't actually have the flu," says Paul Lachance, Ph.D., a nutrition professor at Rutgers University. "They literally get sick from their diet."

63. Hold off for six months. According to a researcher for the U.S. Department of Agriculture (USDA), people who learn to eliminate excess fat tend to lose their craving for it over time. In other words, six months from now you won't even miss those kielbasa sandwiches.

64. Know your weaknesses. Your problem may not be that you eat too much of everything, but that you have a weakness for certain fattening foods—ice cream, chocolate, pastry, potato chips. Once you've identified your problem foods, you'll find it easier to resist them and reward yourself in other ways.

65. Treat yourself. Low-fat or nonfat frozen yogurt, vanilla wafers (19 calories each versus 90 calories for some premium chocolate-chip cookies), popcorn, and fruit are especially good. When none of your diet foods stimulates your taste buds, you may give in when a more tempting snack comes your way.

66. Tap into partner power. Having support at home, especially from your partner, makes all the difference. One study found that one of the most important success factors for dieters was involvement by other family members, especially a spouse.

Beating Binges

67. HALT binges. Don't get too *H*ungry, *A*ngry, *L*onely, or *T*ired. Any one of these feelings could spark a binge. Employed by many counseling groups such as Overeaters Anonymous, this little acronym can remind you to take care of yourself.

68. Eat three square meals a day. This will keep you from getting hungry and can prevent binge eating, say experts in the field of eating disorders.

69. Address your anger. Anger is a signal that someone is violating an important standard of yours, and it can lead to overeating. To cool down the emotion, think of how you can avoid future violations. For instance, you might request that your colleagues move their loud conversations away from your desk. If you can't prevent a recurrence, think of a better response, such as blowing off

steam with exercise. And reevaluate your standards—
maybe you're expecting too much.

70. Stay in touch. Loneliness is a signal that you
need a particular kind of contact with people. Figure out
what kind of contact you need and with whom, and then
initiate that contact.

71. Sleep tight. Many people turn to food as a pick-
me-up when they're running ragged. Make sure you get a
full night's sleep, and you won't get so tired.

How to Harness the Hungries

72. "Ruin" your appetite. When the munchies hit,
try gargling with mouthwash instead of eating, advises
personal trainer Doug Larson. "You just don't feel like
eating when your mouth is fresh and clean," says Larson,
who keeps a bottle of mouthwash in his refrigerator. Use
one without alcohol.

73. Use a souped-up appetite suppressant. Next
time you're hungry, try a bowl of tomato soup to fill you
up. In a study of how goods satisfy, 12 subjects who had
a tomato soup appetizer ate less of a second course than
subjects who ate equal calories of either cantaloupe slices
or cheese on crackers.

74. Snuff out your hunger. To stifle your appetite,
have a high-protein snack about 20 minutes before the
main course, recommends Steven R. Peikin, M.D., director
of gastrointestinal nutrition at Thomas Jefferson University
Hospital in Philadelphia and author of *The Feel Full Diet.*
Suggestions include 2 tablespoons of peanut butter on a
celery stick, a 4-ounce can of water-packed tuna, or 2
ounces of low-fat mozzarella cheese.

75. Derail that craving. When the urge to eat strikes, try one of these strategies.

• Go for a walk.
• Brush your teeth before eating (the sweetness may retard hunger, and you may feel less like gumming up the works with food).
• Wait awhile before giving in to your craving—maybe you'll decide it's not worth it.
• If you simply must have that 5th Avenue bar, eat half and throw away the rest.

Fit Bits and Exercise Tips

76. Use it or lose it in three months. Muscular strength gained in weight training lasts for about 12 weeks after workouts are stopped or reduced, concludes a study at the University of Florida's Center for Exercise Sciences. By the end of that period, subjects had lost 68 percent of the strength they had gained during training.

77. Don't take a vacation from your workouts. Nearly 1,000 YMCAs across the country are allowing members of one facility to attend others while traveling. The AWAY program—an acronym for Always Welcome At YMCAs—allows full-privilege members to attend YMCA facilities in other towns free of charge or at a reduced rate. What's needed is a special sticker for your membership card, which is available—along with a directory of Ys participating in AWAY—at any member YMCA facility.

78. Workouts too much work? It could be that you're iron-deficient. Studies by USDA researchers show that women who showed signs of iron deficiency, but weren't anemic, used less oxygen during exercise and accumulated more lactate, which causes that "lead in the legs" feeling. Result: A more sluggish feeling during exercise. Iron deficiency is a big problem for women. (They lose considerable amounts during menstruation.) Research shows that nearly 80 percent of women consume less than the RDA of 15 milligrams. (Men should consume 10 milligrams daily.) Good sources include organ meats, spinach, and kale.

79. Be an early exercise bird. A study by the Southwest Health Institute in Phoenix found that three of four people who are morning exercisers continued their workouts one year later. By comparison, only half of midday exercisers and one in four evening exercisers did. Theory: Excuses to not exercise are more likely to occur as the day progresses.

80. Take yourself for a walk. Of the various forms of exercise, walking stands out. It's easiest to do and requires no special equipment. Walking doesn't burn the calories off as fast as running does—running burns off about 20 percent more—but the novice exerciser can usually walk farther than he can run. A 150-pound man walking at a good clip—roughly 4 miles per hour—for 45 minutes three times a week will drop about 18 pounds in a year, according to John C. Wolf, D.O., an associate professor of family medicine at the College of Osteopathic Medicine, Ohio University, in Athens, Ohio.

81. Think 20 plus: The magic number for burning fat. Studies show that the rate of fat burning increases for all types of exercise after the first 20 minutes. The average walker burns about 200 calories on a brisk 20-minute walk, and roughly half those calories come from fat. After 20 minutes, the rate of fat calories burned escalates to about 70 percent, according to Tom R. Thomas, Ph.D., from the exercise physiology laboratory at the University of Missouri.

82. Get out in the cold. Although cold weather discourages most of us from exercising, winter is one of the best times to get out and put your body through its paces. In the cold, your body needs to burn more calories to maintain its normal temperature.

83. Ski yourself skinny. Cross-country skiing is one of the best calorie-burners on the books, at about 700 calories per hour for a 150- to 160-pound man.

84. Lift weight and lose fat. When you diet, you lose fat—and muscle along with it. That's also true of diet coupled with aerobic exercise. But circuit weight training may help you lose more fat while retaining more muscle. Researchers at Atlanta's Emory University found that test subjects who engaged in circuit weight training while dieting had 85 percent of their weight loss as fat—13 percent more than dieters who did aerobics.

85. Turn on the tunes. Music lowers perceptions of fatigue and pain, allowing you to push harder with less apparent effort, according to research at Ohio State University. But that's not all: Music also "enhances your rapport with your body," says Kenneth Bruscia, Ph.D., a music therapy professor at Temple University. "It increases endurance, regulates breathing rates, and establishes a mood for physical activity."

86. Learn how to adapt. Overtraining may actually put a damper on your weight-loss program. Losing weight is hard on the body, which must continually adapt to the increase in exercise and the decrease in calories. Eventually, the body may reach a point where it fights back by lowering its metabolism. You plateau and stop losing weight. If this happens to you, decrease your exercise regimen to give your body a chance to adjust.

87. When to eat and run. If you're more than 30 percent above your ideal weight, exercising before a meal burns more calories. If you're less than 30 percent above your ideal weight, exercising after eating burns more calories.

88. Don't knock yourself out. A fairly long session of moderate excercise burns more fat than a short session of intense exercise, says fitness expert Peter Francis, Ph.D., of San Diego State University. You don't need to work yourself into an aerobic frenzy, just keep up a comfortable pace for a longer period.

89. Put some fun in your fitness. If jogging bores you, don't jog, advises Dr. Hagerman. "Recreational athletes always ask, 'Can I watch TV? Can I read? Can I listen to my tapes?' " he says. "Do what you must to make exercise more pleasurable."

Sneak Exercise into Your Life

90. Pedal places. Take your bike, not your car, when doing errands. You'll burn off a lot more calories, and you might even find errands more enjoyable when you tackle them by bicycle.

91. Step up to slim down. Take the stairs instead of the elevator. Stair climbing burns more calories than jogging and cycling.

92. Get on your feet. Standing burns more calories than sitting, so try to stay on your feet. If you have a sit-down job, stand up while talking on the phone, for instance.

CHAPTER

6

GREAT-TASTING LEAN RECIPES: THE PERFECT FORMULA FOR TRIMMING DOWN TO SIZE

◆

You don't have to cut out flavor to peel off the pounds. *Prevention*'s taste-testers agree: Low-fat cuisine can be downright delicious!

To give you a sampling of what's out there, here's a collection of dishes that taste-testers considered this year's best. They're healthy, they're low in calories and fat, and most important, they taste great.

Creole Spinach Salad

    1 pound fresh spinach, cleaned, with tough stems removed
    1 medium red onion, thinly sliced
    4 slices whole wheat bread, toasted and cubed
    2 tablespoons roasted pecans, finely chopped
    ¼ cup nonfat yogurt
    ¼ cup prepared mustard
    2 tablespoons lemon juice
    2 tablespoons balsamic vinegar
    1 teaspoon Creole Seasoning*
      hot-pepper sauce, to taste
      ground white pepper, to taste
    ¼ cup defatted chicken stock

In a large bowl, toss together the spinach, onions, bread cubes, and pecans.

Place the yogurt, mustard, lemon juice, vinegar, Creole Seasoning, hot-pepper sauce, and white pepper in a blender and process on high for 1 minute. With the blender running, slowly pour in the stock.

* To make Creole Seasoning, combine 2½ tablespoons paprika, 2 tablespoons dried garlic or garlic powder, 2 tablespoons black pepper, 1 tablespoon red pepper, 1 tablespoon dried thyme, 1 tablespoon dried oregano, and 1 tablespoon dried onions or onion powder in a small bowl. Keep leftover seasoning in a tightly sealed jar in a cool, dry place.

Pour the dressing over the salad. Toss well to combine.

4 servings. Per serving: 149 calories, 4.1 grams fat (25 percent of calories), 4 grams dietary fiber

Squash Soup

1 butternut squash (about 6 pounds), quartered and seeded
5½ cups stock
2 medium onions, chopped
3 stalks celery, thinly sliced
½ teaspoon dried sage or 1 teaspoon minced fresh sage
1 tablespoon ground coriander
1 tablespoon honey
1 teaspoon ground cumin

Steam the squash over boiling water until tender. Set aside until cool enough to handle. Scoop the flesh from the shell and mash well. You should have about 4 cups of squash. Set aside.

In a 3-quart saucepan, combine the stock, onions, celery, and sage. Bring to a boil, then reduce the heat and simmer for 20 minutes, or until the vegetables are tender.

Add the squash, coriander, honey, and cumin. Place in a blender and process on medium (working in batches) until smooth. Return the soup to the pan and simmer for 15 minutes.

4 to 5 servings. Per serving: 72 calories, 1 gram fat (12.5 percent of calories), 2 grams dietary fiber

Apricot and Rice Muffins

1½ cups unbleached flour
⅔ cup whole wheat flour
⅓ cup rice bran
1 tablespoon baking powder
1 teaspoon ground cinnamon
1 cup cooked short-grain brown rice
1½ cups diced dried apricots
½ cup raisins
½ cup diced prunes
¼ cup chopped walnuts
1 cup nonfat yogurt
⅔ cup maple syrup
¼ cup vegetable oil
1 egg, lightly beaten, or ¼ cup egg substitute

In a large bowl, combine the flours, rice bran, baking powder, and cinnamon. Stir in the rice, apricots, raisins, prunes, and walnuts.

In a small bowl, whisk together the yogurt, maple syrup, oil, and egg. Pour over the dry ingredients, and carefully fold together until just moistened. Do not overmix.

Line 18 muffin cups with paper liners. Divide the batter among the cups, filling almost to the top. Bake at 350°F for 45 minutes, or until the edges and tops begin to brown.

18 muffins. Per muffin: 192 calories, 5 grams fat (23 percent of calories), 2.7 grams dietary fiber

Spicy Black Beans

   1 cup dried black beans, soaked overnight
   ½ cup chopped fresh basil
   1 small hot chili pepper, minced, with seeds
      removed
   1 tablespoon olive oil
   2 cloves garlic, minced

Drain the beans and place them in a 2-quart saucepan with water to cover. Bring to a boil, then reduce the heat, cover loosely, and simmer until tender, about 1 hour. Drain, reserving the liquid.

Return the beans to the saucepan. Add the basil, pepper, oil, garlic, and enough of the reserved liquid to cover.

Bring to a boil, reduce the heat, and simmer for 30 minutes, or until the beans are tender and the liquid is thick.

4 servings. Per serving: 200 calories, 4.1 grams fat (18 percent of calories), 5.1 grams dietary fiber

NOTE: This recipe makes about 2 cups of cooked beans. You can easily double it to make 4 servings of the Beans and Rice Combo Plate (see page 150).

Beans and Rice Combo Plate

1 cup Spicy Black Beans (see page 149)
1 cup cooked brown rice
1 ounce low-fat cheddar cheese, shredded
2 tablespoons salsa
2 tablespoons nonfat yogurt
1 tablespoon minced sweet red pepper
1 tablespoon minced onion
1 tablespoon shredded lettuce
1 tablespoon minced fresh coriander

Serve the beans and rice topped with the cheddar, salsa, yogurt, red pepper, onions, lettuce, and coriander.

1 serving. Per serving: 510 calories, 7.1 grams fat (12 percent of calories), 10.2 grams dietary fiber

Poached Salmon with Citrus Relish

Citrus relish
1 medium pink grapefruit
1 medium navel orange
1 medium lemon
½ cup shredded onion
¼ cup diced sweet red pepper
1 tablespoon minced fresh chervil
1 teaspoon olive oil
1 teaspoon honey
   black pepper, to taste

Salmon

1 pound filleted salmon
1 pound green beans, cleaned and trimmed
1 tablespoon olive oil
1 tablespoon rice-wine vinegar or cider vinegar
   minced fresh cilantro or snipped chives for
   garnish
4 slices Italian bread

To make the citrus relish: Peel the grapefruit,
orange, and lemon with a knife. Cut sections away from
the membranes. Squeeze juice from the membranes and
the pulp clinging to them, and reserve ¼ cup.

Place the fruit in a large bowl with the onions, peppers, and chervil. Drizzle with oil and honey and sprinkle
with pepper. Toss to combine. Set aside.

To make the salmon: Cut the fish crosswise into 12
equal medallions. Steam over boiling water until cooked
through, about 4 minutes. Chill.

Blanch the beans in boiling water until bright green,
about 1 minute. Drain.

In a wok or large skillet, bring the reserved juice,
the oil, and the vinegar to a boil. Add the beans and toss
until coated.

Arrange three slices of salmon in a fan shape on
each dinner plate. Spoon on the citrus relish. Divide
beans among plates. Garnish with cilantro or chives.
Serve warm with Italian bread.

*4 servings. Per serving: 359 calories (30 percent
from fat), 3.5 grams dietary fiber.*

Pasta with Zucchini and Fresh Tomatoes

4 small zucchinis (about 1 pound)
2 tablespoons lemon juice
3 cloves garlic, minced
1 teaspoon olive oil
2 medium onions, thinly sliced and separated into rings
1 tablespoon vinegar
3 large ripe tomatoes, thinly sliced
1/4 cup minced fresh basil
1 tablespoon minced fresh parsley
1/2 teaspoon crushed red pepper
1 pound ziti

Halve the zucchinis and slice into 1/2-inch sections. Place in a large bowl, add the lemon juice, and toss. Set aside.

Spray a large nonstick skillet with no-stick cooking spray. Sauté the garlic in the oil over medium-high heat for 1 minute, stirring constantly. Don't let it burn. Add the zucchini, onions, and vinegar. Cook for 3 to 4 minutes.

Add the tomatoes, basil, parsley, and pepper. Toss to blend. Cover the pan, reduce the heat, and simmer until the zucchini is tender, about 5 to 7 minutes.

Meanwhile, bring a large pot of water to a boil. Add the ziti and cook until just tender. Drain and place in a large shallow bowl. Spoon the zucchini mixture over it. Serve immediately. .

6 servings. Per serving: 330 calories, 2.7 grams fat (6 percent of calories), 4.3 grams dietary fiber

Pizza Dough

    1 cup lukewarm water
    1 package active dry yeast
    ⅛ teaspoon salt
    2 cups unbleached flour
    1½ cups whole wheat flour

In a large bowl, combine the water, yeast, and salt.
Stir and allow to proof for 5 minutes or until foamy. Stir
in the unbleached flour and mix with a wooden spoon
until smooth. Gradually add the whole wheat flour to
form a soft dough.

Turn the dough out onto a lightly floured surface
and knead until smooth, about 8 minutes.

Place the dough in a large nonstick pan, cover with
a towel, and set in a warm, draft-free place to rise until
doubled in bulk, about 1½ to 2 hours.

Punch down the dough and knead for 2 minutes.
Return to the pan. Cover and let rise for 1 hour. At this
point, the dough is ready to be rolled out.

*1 crust; 4 servings. Per serving: 383 calories,
1.3 grams fat (3 percent of calories), 7.9 grams dietary
fiber*

NOTE: Pizza must be baked in an intensely hot oven, about 450° to
500°F. It is also best if baked directly on hot unglazed ceramic tiles or
a pizza stone. Place the tiles or stone in the oven before preheating
so they're hot when the pizza is ready to be baked.

Roasted Eggplant and Garlic Pizza

    Pizza Dough (see page 153)
1 pound eggplant
1 head garlic, cloves peeled
1 teaspoon minced fresh thyme
1 teaspoon minced fresh rosemary
1 onion, thinly sliced and separated into rings
¼ cup defatted stock
1 tablespoon minced fresh parsley
⅛ teaspoon ground black pepper

On a cookie sheet or pizza tin, roll the dough into a circle about 12 to 14 inches in diameter. Cover with plastic wrap and set aside.

Cut the eggplant in half lengthwise. Place, cut side down, on a nonstick baking sheet. Place the garlic, thyme, and rosemary on a square of foil. Fold to enclose the herbs completely, then crimp and seal the packet. Place on the baking sheet with the eggplant. Bake at 450°F for 20 to 30 minutes. Remove from the oven and set aside to cool. Keep garlic mixture in foil.

In a large nonstick skillet, sauté the onions in the stock, stirring occasionally, until translucent, about 5 to 7 minutes. Set aside.

When the eggplant is cool enough to handle, gently peel the skin, leaving the flesh intact. With a sharp knife, cut the flesh into thin slices.

Uncover the crust and arrange half of the eggplant and half of the garlic mixture over the crust. Spread with the onions. Arrange the remaining eggplant and garlic mixture over the top. Sprinkle with the parsley and pepper.

Bake at 450° to 500°F for about 15 minutes, or until the crust is browned and crisp.

4 servings. Per serving: 439 calories, 1.5 grams fat (3 percent of calories), 8.5 grams dietary fiber

Delicious Simple Chicken

3 boneless, skinless chicken breasts, split
2 teaspoons olive oil
¼ cup minced fresh herbs
3 cloves garlic, minced

Trim the chicken of all visible fat. Place the pieces between sheets of wax paper and use a mallet to pound to an even thickness. Rub each piece with oil.

Combine the herbs and garlic to make a paste. Rub the paste onto all sides of the chicken. Cover and refrigerate for 30 minutes.

Place each breast on a large sheet of foil, then fold the foil to make a tightly sealed packet. Place the packets directly on the oven rack and bake at 400°F for 7 to 10 minutes.

4 to 6 servings. Per serving: 152 calories, 3.8 grams fat (23 percent of calories)

NOTE: To make chicken burritos, cut the chicken into chunks or thin strips. Wrap in flour tortillas and top with your choice of salsa, nonfat yogurt, shredded lettuce, or other chopped vegetables.

Sunshine Fruit Shake

    1 cup skim milk
    ½ frozen banana, coarsely chopped
    ½ frozen persimmon, coarsely chopped, seeds
        removed
    1 date or fig, chopped
    1 tablespoon rolled oats or bran flakes
    1 tablespoon instant nonfat dry milk
        pinch of ground cinnamon

Place the milk, banana, persimmon, and date or fig in a blender. Blend on medium speed for about 10 seconds.

Add the oats or bran flakes and dry milk to the mixture. Blend for 15 seconds, or until smooth. Pour into a glass and sprinkle with the cinnamon.

1 serving. Per serving: 256 calories, 1.3 grams fat (4 percent of calories), 1.9 grams dietary fiber

Banana-Strawberry Whip

    1 frozen banana, partially defrosted
    4 fresh strawberries
    ⅓ teaspoon honey
    8 teaspoons soy fiber powder
    1 cup skim milk

Place ingredients in a blender and whip to the desired consistency.

2 cups.

NOTE: The soy fiber powder in this drink provides 16 grams of dietary fiber.

Berry Crisp

 3 cups mixed fresh or frozen berries
 2 tablespoons lemon juice
 ½ cup whole wheat pastry flour
 ½ cup toasted rolled oats
 ½ teaspoon ground cinnamon
 ¼ cup maple syrup

Coat a 9-inch glass pie plate with nonstick spray.
Add the berries and lemon juice. Toss to combine. Be
careful not to bruise the berries.

In a small bowl, stir together the flour, oats, and
cinnamon. Add the maple syrup and stir with a fork until
crumbly. Sprinkle over the berries and cover the dish
with foil. Bake at 400°F until the berries are bubbly,
about 20 minutes. Remove the foil and bake for about
5 minutes more, or until the crust is medium brown.

*8 servings. Per serving: 107 calories, 0.7 grams fat
(6 percent of calories), 4.1 grams dietary fiber*

CHAPTER

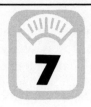

7

PROFILES OF
WINNERS AT LOSING

Each year *Prevention* gets scores of letters from happy readers telling their weight-loss success stories. Many are so inspiring that we wish more could be repeated here. Unfortunately, space doesn't permit.

Here are six stories of astounding victory over weight. Motivating and inspiring, each story reveals the strategies that made these people winners at *losing.* Each of them is genuine, living proof that lifelong weight control is more than a pipe dream.

Sick and Tired of Being Obese

Marlin Groff had battled obesity most of his life. But this manager of an answering-service and accounting firm in Akron, Pennsylvania, found the war had taken a nasty turn. At 6 feet, 2 inches and 427 pounds, his cholesterol level, blood pressure, and heart rate were all dangerously high. And because of a life-threatening sleep disorder caused by his weight, Marlin needed surgery to have a breathing tube implanted in his throat. Finally, though, he spent two years developing his own personal plan for weight loss—and followed it for the next 39 months. Now a svelte 187 pounds, Marlin has recovered his health and says he has everything to live for.

"I was a really skinny kid until I was eight years old. Then, all of a sudden, I started gaining weight. My parents were moderately overweight, so I figured I was destined to be overweight, too.

"I weighed about 200 pounds my freshman year in high school and 285 when I graduated. At 6 feet, 2 inches tall, I can carry a little more weight than some people. But when I hit 40 years old, I started to add even more weight steadily. I didn't pay much attention, and it just kept climbing. Then when I was 44, I started having troublesome sleep disturbances.

"A specialist diagnosed my problem as sleep apnea,

a condition in which you actually stop breathing. It was caused by the excess weight obstructing my windpipe. My case was so severe that my heart would actually stop beating, and when it restarted, the restart actually kicked me out of bed.

"The doctor told me I had to have a tracheostomy. A hole would be cut in my throat and a breathing tube inserted. They told me my case was so severe that if I didn't have the surgery soon, I would probably die in my sleep.

"The thought of having a tube put in my throat was devastating. But I knew I had no choice, and I went along with it.

"The night before my surgery, they had to take me downstairs to the hospital freight room to weigh me. They put me on the scale and told me I weighed 427 pounds. I was stunned.

"After the surgery I spent a lot of time feeling sorry for myself. I hated the tube in my throat. I hated myself because I was so fat. I wallowed in self-pity for a long time.

"About six months after the surgery I lost my job because my company went bankrupt. It took ten months to find a new job. It seemed like nobody wanted to hire me. I'm sure it was because of the weight and the tracheostomy. I became severely depressed."

A Crucial Moment

"I had reached the point where I had nothing to live for except my family. I wanted to get professional help, but being out of work, I just couldn't afford it. Then I was watching a talk show one night, and I saw a doctor who spoke about a high-carbohydrate, low-fat diet for losing weight.

"He said you can eat more calories if they come from carbohydrates instead of fats. This caught my interest because whenever I had tried to lose weight before, it was always on a 1,000- or 1,200-calorie diet. I would lose 50 or 60 pounds, but I would be starving, so I couldn't stay on it. It was a cycle I went through over and over throughout my adult life.

"So I went to the library and started reading everything I could on carbohydrates, fats, and protein, and also behavior modification. That was in the fall of 1986.

"I started putting down on paper what I thought might work for me, taking into consideration my personal food preferences. I kept reading, trying to find out which foods would be the most effective for me to focus on.

"I started out with 1,800 calories a day (down from around 4,000 calories a day at 427 pounds), with only 20 percent of those calories coming from fat.

"I took it up to 2,200 calories several times because I was losing a little faster than my doctor thought was best—between 3 and 4 pounds a week. Although I had a lot of weight to lose, I didn't want to lose it too quickly. I was very concerned about losing muscle, particularly heart muscle, because I was physically unable to exercise in the beginning.

"I also figured out which foods I absolutely shouldn't eat and how I could avoid them. I was a potato chip freak, for example. So I used a book I found in the library on aversion therapy to overcome the problem. I simply imagined a bowl of potato chips in front of me and pretended I saw green worms growing all over them.

"Then I visualized myself eating them, green worms and all. I practiced this for about a month. It worked. I haven't given in to potato chips since. Instead, once a month I prove my new control to myself by eating just one.

"I cut fat everywhere I could. I used only 1 teaspoon of margarine a day. And I really restricted my meat intake. I could have 6 ounces of fish, but if I was eating poultry or red meat, 3 or 4 ounces was the most I could have and keep the meal at the 20 percent level. I seldom ate red meat, though, and I increased my intake of complex carbohydrates, such as whole grains, fruit, and vegetables.

"I kept a food diary for the first 18 months. Every night I totaled the number of calories I'd eaten for the day. Of course, I cheated occasionally. But if I had 1,850 calories one day, I would make sure to have only 1,750 the next."

The Final Stretch

"When I had lost 130 pounds, a sleep study test showed that the sleep apnea was gone and the doctors were able to remove the breathing tube in my throat.

"I could have stopped losing weight at that point. But I realized that I had finally found a way to lose weight and keep it off. I decided to go all the way.

"My ultimate goal was to get down to 187 pounds. But I set small goals along the way. First I tried to get under 400, then under 350, then under 300.

"After that, I set my goals in 25-pound increments. There were plateau periods when I didn't lose anything for two weeks at a time, but then I would lose 4 or 5 pounds again.

"After I had lost 40 pounds, I started walking. I had bad arthritis in both of my knees, and walking was really a chore at first. I could barely get out of chairs without pain. I started out walking ¾ mile and built it up gradually to 4 miles. I tried to walk every day. The arthritis got better and better, and I kept losing weight.

"My wife, Gale, and I walk almost all year round in all kinds of weather. I started using an exercise bike, too. I now ride between 8 and 16 miles each day. I also began doing 20 to 30 minutes of calisthenics each day, and lifting weights."

Free from Fat, at Last!

"Needless to say, now that I'm down to 187 pounds my whole life has changed. The doctor has reduced my blood pressure and heart rate medication to about one-third of what I took before. My cholesterol dropped from 265 to 147. And my triglycerides dropped down to normal, too. My waist size went from 66 to 36. It's like half a person is completely gone.

"Just to be able to walk into a clothing store and go to the regular-size rack to pick out clothes is an incredible feeling. For the first time, I honestly feel like the man I always wanted to be.

"Recently I had some excess abdominal skin removed—7 pounds of it! My whole life I always wanted to be a thin person, and now I am! That alone has made all of this worthwhile."

No More "Diets," Just Common Sense

To hear 54-year-old office manager Roberta Mulliner talk about the 95 pounds she lost, you almost have to wonder how she did it. Part of her "wanted to fail," she says: the part that blamed her weight on a plump family tree. And the part that "would kill" for a good jelly doughnut or an all-you-can-eat breakfast at the local fire hall. But with a pinch of smarter eating and an armload of exercise, Roberta discovered that her weight problem wasn't in her genes, after all. It was only in her jeans, which she was able to shrink from jumbo to genteel.

"When you grow up with giants, you tend not to notice that you're becoming one yourself. Both of my parents were on the heavy side and my brother, too. We never thought of each other as fat, however. Just big-boned. All part of being German, we figured.

"But it's tough to hold on to a belief like that when, at 5 feet, 9 inches and 265 pounds, you start working at a company that has its own gym and its own health-food cafeteria, and you suddenly find yourself surrounded by people who are super-fit and practically bouncing off the

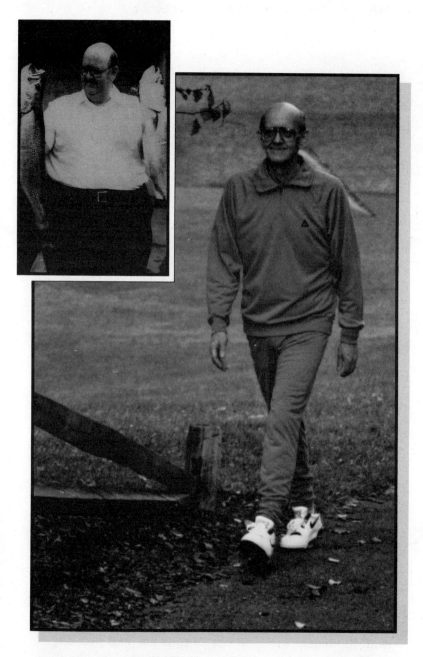

Marlin Groff shed 240 pounds in 39 months. His successful strategies included starting a low-fat, high-carbohydrate diet, walking, riding an exercise bike, and strength training.

walls with energy. I suddenly felt like Gulliver among the Lilliputians.

"I was able to hide behind my heavy family tree theory for a few years before a voice inside me started whispering 'coward'. The voice was saying 'find out once and for all if your weight problem is really etched in genetic stone, and if it is (which in a way I hoped it was), learn to live with it guilt-free!'

"At 53 I figured I finally owed it to myself to find the truth. I decided to give myself a good year. I wasn't going to rush it or try anything gimmicky because I'd already been down that path too many times. I was going to try it right this time—slow and steady, and with exercise as my guiding light. I had been reading a lot and I knew that exercise was important not just for burning calories, but also for preventing loss of muscle tissue and for keeping the metabolism up. And for keeping the spirits up, too. On so many diets I had tried, what finally would do me in was depression. My spirits would sink so low that my self-esteem would follow. And bingo, I'd be into the maple-walnut ice cream with a tablespoon."

The Key Element: Exercise

"I had always thought of myself as a very clumsy kid, and for good reason, I guess, so I was not out to set any records. I just decided to get an hour of exercise every day. I started walking in the mornings before work, a few blocks at first, and then a few more. Within a few months I was up to a couple of miles and actually liking it!

"But I wanted to keep good muscle tone all over my body, not just in my legs, so I started using the weight machines at the company gym. Three days a week I'd work with the machines for about 40 minutes, and in a circuit fashion, going from machine to machine with about 35 seconds of aerobics, such as walking or stationary bike riding, in between. I actually got to enjoy that, too. Had there been an athlete hiding inside my 'clumsy' body all these years after all? I began to wonder. Exercise had always been a dirty word to me, but now it was my gospel. On the days I didn't do circuits I added two aerobics classes a week to my schedule to give me even more variety, and on weekends I walked.

"And I loved the results I was getting, too. People at work started complimenting me on my appearance after just a few months, and it felt great. It felt great to go shopping for new clothes, too. My dress sizes were falling faster than the stock market—eventually to a 12 all the way from a 22. My blood pressure was heading downward, too—from 150/110 to 120/80.

"The only thing on the rise was my self-esteem and my energy. I used to pretty much just collapse in front of the TV after dinner, but now I was sewing or running errands or even finding something to clean. Don't let anyone ever tell you exercise poops you out. If you do it right, it revs you up."

Learning to Eat Lean

"Exercise was only half of my strategy, however. In addition to sticking to at least an hour of exercise a day, I was going to declare all-out war on fat. And what really surprised me was that it was easier and tastier than I had thought. It's really amazing how your taste buds adapt. Before long I wasn't missing the fried foods, gravies, or fatty condiments at all. My daughter and husband were squawking a bit, but gradually they started coming my way, too. A typical day's menu for me would go like this:

Lunch: Low-fat yogurt, a piece of fruit, and a rice cake.

Dinner: Pretty much anything I wanted, but nothing fried and no rich sauces, gravies, or butter. Plus, I'd always have two vegetables and a big salad without any dressing. I came to appreciate the fresh tastes, plus it would really fill me up.

Dessert: I've always loved to eat ice cream, so I didn't deprive myself of that pleasure. I would eat the low-fat versions, though, and the low-fat frozen yogurts.

Snacks: I've always been a snacker, too, so I didn't deprive myself of that, either. I'd snack mostly on rice cakes, air-popped popcorn, and vegetable sticks. I think snacks are important. If you enjoy snacking, you should let yourself do it as long as what you snack on is low in fat, calories, and salt. If you resist the urge to snack, I think it comes back to haunt you, and all too often in the form of a binge.

"I stuck to this plan for a year and it's still pretty much the way I continue to eat now. It's nothing too radical, I know, but maybe that's why it worked and why it continues to work. It doesn't feel like a diet."

It Just Gets Easier

"I look back now at all the times I failed at losing weight and I can't believe how stupid I was. If you commit yourself to just two basic principles, you'll lose weight. You just have to increase your exercise and decrease your dietary fat. People see the change in me and say things like, 'You're unbelievable, Roberta. How did you do it? It must have been such a struggle.' But it wasn't a struggle. I'm not going to say I always felt like getting up early enough to get my walk in before work, or that I don't sometimes still long for a jelly doughnut, but on certain occasions I give in. I think one of the reasons I've been successful in my weight loss this time has been that I've learned to give in without going to pieces. Before, I'd make one slip and then just keep on sliding. But now I can enjoy an occasional splurge and put on the brakes. I think it's because I have confidence in knowing that the program I'm on now is the right one. I still have about 15 more pounds I'd like to lose, but I'm in no hurry. Why should I be? I didn't rush the first 95 pounds, so why start now?"

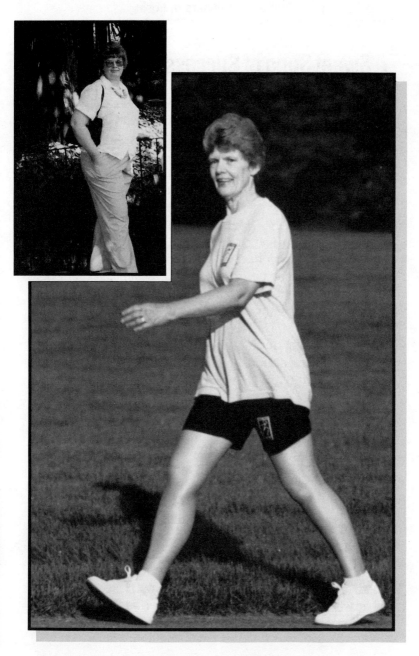

By getting hooked on exercise, cutting fat, and learning to love *healthy* snacks, Roberta Mulliner lost 95 pounds in one year. Now she enjoys greater energy, lower blood pressure, and improved self-esteem.

A Sweet Song of Success

Dianne Anderson hit bottom when her weight and blood pressure went through the roof. At 321 pounds, the 5-foot, 7-inch music teacher from Forest Park, Georgia, was even having trouble on the job—her weight and lack of fitness left her unable to demonstrate proper breathing techniques to her vocal students. But with a winning harmony of smart nutrition, regular exercise, friendly support, and patience, Dianne found her own way to achieve permanent weight loss and make beautiful music once more.

"When I was a child, I was a tomboy, and my vigorous lifestyle prevented me from having a weight problem despite a big appetite. But that all changed as I entered my teens, and especially when I went away to college. My activity level decreased as my poor eating habits increased. I was eating a lot of snack foods that were high in calories and fat, and the pounds kept piling on.

"Eventually, my eating became a form of escape, a world in which I felt secure. But the truth was that every bite was making me less secure. As my weight went up, my self-confidence went down, and I became withdrawn and afraid that people were making fun of me. I wasn't a wallflower—I just flat refused to attend a social activity!

"When I took up teaching, I think my weight even limited the amount of respect I was able to command from my students. And because the excess weight and lack of fitness hampered my ability to breathe properly, it became impossible for me to perform well vocally.

"Of course, my parents and my doctor had encouraged me for years to change, but I didn't seem to have what was needed to accomplish that. I had tried dieting, but the pounds never stayed off."

Getting in Tune with Her Health

"It really was a combination of factors that finally got me to try again. For one thing, my blood pressure went extremely high, and I had to take medication to control it. For the first time I realized that my uncontrolled eating was quite literally killing me. Also, I have a religious belief that our bodies are God's temple, and he expects us to be good stewards and treat them well. But I was abusing my body. I was destroying my own health just because I wanted to eat.

"Then one day a friend of mine, Margie, asked if I would consider going to Weight Watchers with her. I know that took a bunch of courage, because people who knew me knew that I did not talk about my weight to anybody. She stuck her neck out to bring that subject up, and that really affected me. She and I joined Weight Watchers together.

"That type of approach turned out to be much better because it involved accountability—every week I had to weigh in. Every week I found out how well I had followed through on my commitment.

"Also, it was a nutritionally sound program, based on eating normal food in normal environments. Instead of having to buy special foods, I learned how to eat and cook differently. That really made sense to me.

"So gradually I learned how to change my diet. I didn't keep eating the same fat-filled foods. I quit using regular mayonnaise and butter, and I cut down the amount of oil I was using. I replaced regular salad dressings with either oil-free or low-calorie dressings. I cut back on fatty meats, too. I now eat very little pork and beef. Instead I use fresh fish and poultry. I cut fried foods out of my diet almost totally. And I gave up the fatty snack foods.

"I also started to learn how to cook differently. I don't deep-fry chicken any more—even though deep-frying is traditional here in the South. I steam most of my vegetables, and I've learned to steam fish, too. In fact, I became very interested in how I could take a traditional recipe—like my mother's banana pudding—and reduce the butter and sugar or substitute for them.

"By making these types of changes, I started losing

weight right away—8 pounds the first week. But on average I lost about 2 pounds a week the first year.

"Right away I felt better. Just the decision I had made to change gave me a surge in the beginning, but then the support I started getting from my family and friends—even students—kept the surge alive.

"When I had lost about 50 pounds, my friend Margie told me I'd have to exercise as well as diet because I had so much weight to lose. She was a walker, so I started walking, too.

"At first I just walked for an hour. I could get in only about 3 miles (I still weighed about 270 at that time). But I gradually started going faster till I could get in 4 miles. Then I didn't worry about trying to walk any farther; I just started walking faster. So now I still walk 4 miles, but I do it in about 45 minutes. I do that four days a week, and do toning exercises for my abdominal muscles, arms, and thighs on the other days."

Setting the Tempo for a Great Life

"I lost exactly 100 pounds the first year, but only about 30 the second year. In fact, I had a plateau where I lost nothing for about four months. But I knew what I wanted to do, and that my body was having to make adjustments. I clung to the fact that I wasn't going to stop eating the healthy way I was eating—whether I lost weight or not. I was committed to eating that way for the rest of my life.

"The compliments I received also helped keep me going. One of the more humorous ones was told to me by the mother of one of my students. It seems the student had come home with the joyous announcement that, 'Miss A wore a blouse tucked in her skirt today!'

"By the end of 3½ years, I reached my goal of losing 184 pounds. At 137, I'm smaller now than I was in high school. My blood pressure is normal—I haven't had to take medication for three years. My breathing is much im-

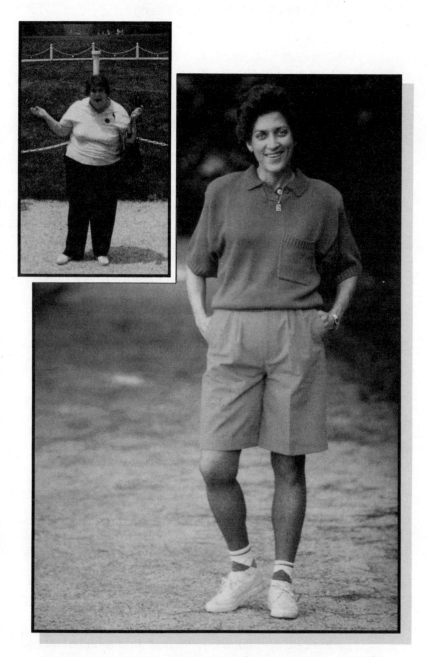

Dianne Anderson improved her overall fitness and her breathing by losing 184 pounds. She did it in 3½ years. "The emotional benefits of losing weight have been phenomenal," she says.

proved, so vocally I'm able to do things now that I couldn't do even in college.

"Of course, my renewed self-confidence helps my performance, too. In fact, the emotional benefits of losing weight have been phenomenal. In the middle of my weight program, I started back to school to work on a master's degree. I know the success I experienced with my weight loss gave me the confidence and courage to go back to college. I finished my master's, and now I'm working on my doctorate—in music education.

"My social life is much more active than it was, too. And there's a fellow that I'm seeing very steadily now. That's a kind of relationship I hadn't enjoyed very often before the weight loss.

"And physically I can do so many things now that I couldn't do before. I was able to go horseback riding last year while on vacation in Colorado—because I didn't weigh more than the horse and he could support my weight! That was the first time since I was a teenager I'd been riding. Recently I entered a 6.2-mile road race in Atlanta and finished in 66 minutes. Part of it I even jogged!"

Sold on Weight Loss

Being 6 feet tall and big-boned helped 51-year-old Dale Warner haul around the 100-plus extra pounds he'd piled on since high school. But when his doctor warned Dale that his weight (300-plus pounds) and the resulting high blood pressure could cause serious heart problems, the Palm Desert, California, salesman listened. By realizing his past mistakes and learning from them, he found his way to permanent weight loss.

Dale took off 80 pounds in the first nine months after visiting his doctor, and another 40 in the following two years. Among the rewards: a new life that includes mountain hiking, wilderness fishing, river rafting, and kayaking.

"In June, 1987, I went for the first physical exam I'd had in eight years. I saw the doctor because I felt dizzy when I bent over to pick things up. I was 48 at the time and thought I was in pretty good shape for someone my age.

"You can imagine my shock when I was told by a very grim-faced doctor that I was well on my way to a heart attack or stroke. He said I had all the symptoms of those silent killers. I was over 100 pounds overweight, my blood pressure was 180/110, my cholesterol was 240, and I had poor lung capacity.

"So my doctor told me to start walking every day. He also gave me a simple list that showed how to exchange fatty, high-calorie foods for healthier fare and told me to come back in six weeks. During the 40-minute drive home, I did some serious thinking. My family had a history of heart disease: A cousin my age had died recently from a heart attack and my father died from a stroke. He had also been overweight. I was scared.

"I had dieted many times before. In fact, once I lost 80 pounds in about a year but gained it back over the next two years. I had made no permanent changes in my lifestyle. I'd diet, then go right back to the same old eating (and beer-drinking) habits. And I had never exercised and dieted at the same time.

"Instead of feeling tied to my past failures, though, I felt hopeful. I realized what was missing in my efforts. The very next day I put those missing pieces into action."

He's Changing His Tastes

"Instead of 'going on a diet,' I incorporated changes in my eating habits that I knew I could stick to permanently. I'd been stopping at a restaurant for breakfast on my way to work to have a three-egg omelet, ham, potatoes, buttered toast, and a large glass of milk. But the next morning I had oatmeal with skim milk. Oddly (and thankfully) enough, it filled me up just fine. I've continued to have oatmeal, or half a cantaloupe, ever since.

"For lunch, I wolfed down steaks or hamburgers and fries. Luckily, most of the restaurants I go to have a salad bar, so now I usually have the biggest salad you've ever seen in your life—dressed lightly with olive oil and vinegar. I also keep greens and vegetables in my refrigerator at the office. A co-worker and I fix ourselves big salads for lunch.

"Dinner now consists mostly of raw vegetables along with some broiled fish. My wife doesn't eat the way I do, but I appreciate that she willingly cooks what I want to eat.

"All this may sound like a hardship, but believe me, it isn't. I've come to enjoy this simple way of eating. Even when I go out with people who are ordering fattening foods, I'm not even tempted. I feel too good to want to eat those foods."

Climbing Higher

"The same morning I chose oatmeal, I also started walking for exercise. That first day I walked for only 10 minutes before I was so exhausted I could barely drag myself back to the house. But I walked again the next morning, and the morning after that, and eventually I started to be energized by the exercise.

"Now I walk into the mountains high above the desert community where I work. There's a 5- and an 8-mile circuit, each with about a 1,200-foot ascent. They are beautiful, sunlit walks. I see things, like little birds, that I had never noticed before because I'd never slowed down enough. I walk, shower, and still open my office by 8 A.M. I sleep so well now that getting up a little earlier doesn't bother me.

"When I returned to my doctor for the six-week checkup, he was impressed with the progress I'd made. After about nine months, I'd lost 80 pounds.

"Over the next two years, another 40 pounds came off, leaving me at about 204. (I'm still about 20 pounds

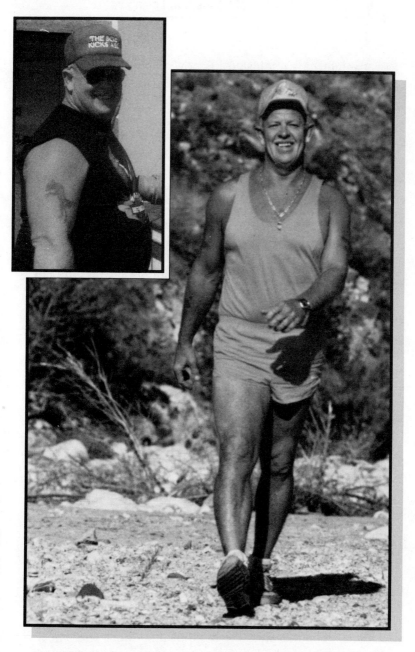

Dale Warner takes a good, long walk every day. That exercise,
along with a low-fat, vegetable-rich diet helped him lose 124 pounds
in 18 months.

overweight.) My cholesterol is now about 142, well within the safe range, and my 'good' HDL cholesterol is high. My blood pressure is much better, too: 130/72. And my resting pulse rate is 50; that of a fit man. At my last visit, my doctor said, 'Walking has changed your life. In fact, I'm sure walking has saved your life, or at least extended it by 20 years.'

"One big change for the better is that I now enjoy outdoor activities. I rarely took vacations because I didn't have the money, and I wasn't fit enough to do very much. Now I have the money, and I want to live long enough to spend it on enjoyable, active vacations. I've gone salmon fishing in Alaska and rafting in the Grand Canyon, and I'm planning a hiking trip in New Zealand. My approach to my vacations mirrors my new approach to life: Staying fit is fun!"

Nursing Herself to Better Health

For more than two decades, operating-room nurse Marjorie Mullaly bounced between fad diets and overeating. She tried diet pills, a liquid diet, and every cockeyed eat-and-lose scheme that popped out of a magazine. Finally, for love of a pair of turquoise sneakers, she was enticed to start walking—and discovered she liked it. She even lost a few pounds. But because she was still eating the same old way, the pounds came back to haunt her.

A gallbladder attack at age 42 finally convinced her to get serious about nutrition as well as workouts. On her own, she developed a program of low-fat meals and exercise that took her from a high of 185 pounds to a svelte 135 that's more compatible with her height of 5 feet, 6 inches. She has shed the big hips and thighs she'd been stuck with since high school. Now she's got confidence, good looks, and endurance. And why not—she's now a marathon runner!

"You name the diet, I've been on it. But as soon as I 'finished' a diet, I started eating just like I used to. And I gained back the pounds I lost plus a few more.

"My size really ballooned when I became pregnant with our first child, Katie. I gained 20 pounds of unnecessary fat during those nine months. And during the years afterward, I kept gaining and losing those same pounds. I tried diet pills. I tried any diet I came across, even the infamous grapefruit diet (in spite of an allergy to citrus fruit).

"The diets wreaked havoc on my health, but they did get the weight off. My problem was keeping it off. Each time I regained, I'd add on a few additional pounds. Slowly, I got heavier and heavier.

"Eight years ago, I hit a new high—170 pounds—far too much for my height. I started to think I was destined to be big."

Time for Herself

"That's when I started to walk. I'd been hearing how it was a great way to lose weight. One day while shopping, I saw a pair of beautiful turquoise sneakers. I decided that I would buy them and walk in them. And I did.

"I loved exercising so much that just a month later, I began to combine running with my walking. Slowly, I built up my time and my distance. In three months, I could run-walk 2 miles. It felt great. I have a very stressful job, and, at the time, I had four children at home. So it was no surprise that my run soon evolved into 'Mother's hour to herself.' I would leave grouchy and come back refreshed.

"Best of all, I began to lose weight. Thirty pounds came off in a matter of months. And it stayed off for a whole year.

"Unfortunately, my road to thinness wasn't a straight one. Because I didn't change my diet while I was running, the weight crept back on during the following year.

"In December 1983, I had a foot operation that sidelined me for a month. By January I had reached my all-time high—185 pounds.

"I was discouraged, but I started to walk and run again. My real turning point, though, didn't come until March. I'd been dieting for almost three months and I was· tired of it. I decided to splurge for a week. In those days, that meant eating rich, fatty, unhealthy foods. The result? I had a dandy gallbladder attack. It was my first one, and when I felt that pain under my ribs, I thought I was dying.

"I was x-rayed at the hospital where I work. I had an inflamed gallbladder and my doctor said an operation was inevitable. I was terrified. But that news turned me around. I immediately went to see a dietitian who offered me some guidelines for a gallbladder diet."

Her Fresh New "Diet"

"That attack was probably the best thing that ever happened to me. The diet I went on was low-fat and high-carbohydrate. And it was delicious! I completely changed the way I ate. I cut out fat and sugar. I started making dishes like steamed vegetables and rice, and pasta.

"I also shifted my main meal from evening to midday. I pared down my dinners to vegetables, a baked potato, or a bowl of oatmeal. I started cooking big batches of food on weekends, freezing portions, and taking them to work every day for lunch.

"I was amazed at how quickly my excess pounds started to drop off. Within seven months I'd lost 50 pounds. The combination of diet and running was a real success. I've kept those 50 pounds off for seven years.

"I loved all the attention I got while I was losing the weight. My kids bragged about me all the time; especially my youngest, Owen, who was eight years old. He would bring his friends over to see how good I looked. Folks at work were very supportive while I was losing, too. They were amazed at how well I was doing. If I didn't see one of them for a week, and then we ran into each other in the hall, I could always count on hearing, 'Oh my gosh, you look great.'

"Of course, it wasn't all easy. Initially, I had trouble cooking separate meals for myself. But as my children have gotten older, they want a sit-down dinner less and less. And my husband, David, has started to eat low-fat foods himself. That's better for him and easier for me. Eating out was a problem, too. Our church has lots of suppers I'd like to attend, but I won't eat that kind of food. Fortunately, we found some restaurants nearby that serve some low-fat entrées."

Crossing the Finish Line to a Better Life

I'm stronger and happier now than ever. Losing weight has done wonderful things for me. I've gained confidence and matured. I never get sick anymore. When I was heavier, I used to get colds all the time and even had pneumonia twice.

"I'm really happy with how I look now, too. It's actually fun to shop for clothes since I've gone from a size 18 to a size 12. I can even share clothes with my youngest daughter, Midge. Sarah and Katie, the older ones, are away at college, or I'd share with them, too.

"My whole look has changed. I got braces, so now my smile is as nice as my figure. And this year I got a perm and changed my hair color. Now that I'm happier with how I look, I have the courage to experiment and try new things.

"The most amazing change since I lost the weight? Believe it or not, I've actually completed two marathons. I ran the first one three years ago, and the second just this year. It took me three years to forget how much the first one hurt. But the sense of accomplishment was great enough that I want to do it again. Next year might be the year that I break my record.

"I know for sure that next year I'll still be eating low-

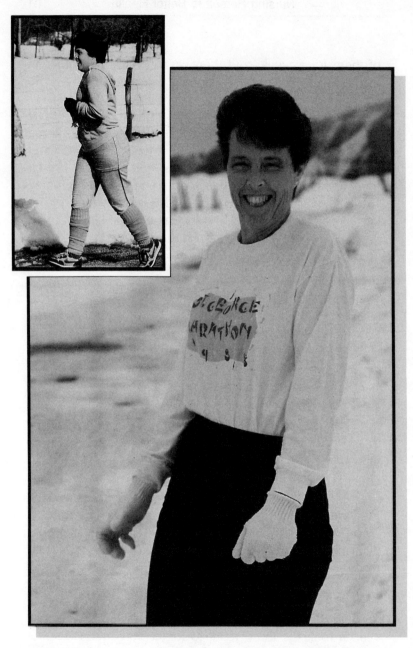

With a weight loss of 50 pounds, Marjorie Mullaly has increased her stamina and decreased her stress. "I'm stronger and happier now than ever," she says.

fat food and I'll still be thin. And I'm going to do the marathon again. I know I can do it."

A Man Who Saved His Own Life

Forty-nine-year-old Howard Bennett had been heavy since he was a child. But a little over two years ago, when at 6 feet, 2 inches, he surpassed 500 pounds, a doctor told him his weight was killing him. Then Howard staged a fight for his life. In 2½ years, he's lost 340 pounds.

"When I was 11 years old, my family moved to Florida. I don't know whether it was the change to Southern-style cooking or my depression over moving that did it. But that was when I started putting on weight. I remember in 1956, my dad, my brother, and I were all the same weight—220 pounds. I was only 14 years old then. I was very self-conscious about my weight, and it kept me from doing a lot of things as I was growing up. I never went to the prom or to dances or ball games.

"By the time I was 42, I weighed 380 pounds. I had moved back to Utah and was working for the Utah Transit Authority. One day I fell off a bus and hurt my back. That really started my weight gain. I had a herniated disk, and osteoporosis developed; I was unable to exercise for two years. I just ate and ate, and kept gaining and gaining.

"I never went to the doctor, but because of my back problem, I was forced to see one about 2½ years ago. I was in bad shape. My blood pressure was high—180/105—and my cholesterol was on the high side at 210. I suffered from sleep apnea, and had developed Type-II diabetes (the kind excess weight can cause). I had edema in my legs, and my feet were so swollen I couldn't even get socks on, let alone shoes. I had to buy moccasins with laces around the toes and undo the laces so my feet would fit in.

"I had reached 530 pounds. The doctor told me I was going to be dead in six months if I didn't get some weight off. It really hit me: I just had to lose weight this time."

Diet Redesign

"I knew what kind of task it was going to be because I'd already been on almost every diet I'd heard of. I would lose weight, but whenever I went off the diets, I'd gain it back, plus a few extra pounds.

"But this time I was better prepared. My dad had gotten me a subscription to *Prevention* magazine for Christmas, and I knew from reading it that dieting often doesn't work. I knew I would have to change my lifestyle and my habits to lose weight. I started by cutting all fats out of my diet and limiting my intake of sugar.

"That in itself changed my diet in a big way. I used to eat a giant bowl of oyster stew for dinner—2 quarts at a sitting. Or I'd eat a couple of hamburgers or hot dogs, or packs of crackers. I liked anything with a lot of cheese on it. I ate a lot of red meat.

"But since I started my low-fat regimen, if I eat any meat, it's chicken baked without the skin. I eat fish two or three times a week, and plain tuna packed in water, not oil. I used to eat it mixed with salad dressing on a sandwich.

"In the first six months after I saw the doctor, I lost about 130 pounds just by watching what I ate. When you're that heavy, weight comes off pretty fast, even without exercise. My weight was still coming down, but so was my mood. I got to feeling really depressed. I guess I was missing the comfort that food used to give me.

"Then I read in *Prevention* about a man who said that walking helped alleviate his depression. I decided to give walking a try."

One Step at a Time

"When I was at my heaviest, I wasn't even able to balance in the shower. I had to have bars built around the bathtub to hold on to while my wife washed me.

"So beginning a walking regimen wasn't easy. At the outset, I had to use a walker just to move around; the drive-

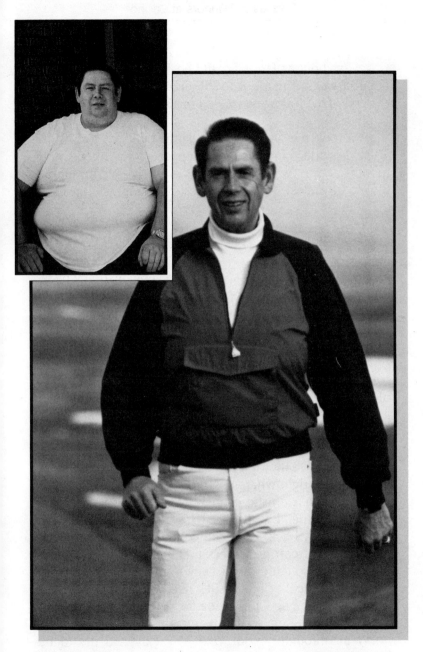

Weighing in 340 pounds *lighter* than he was before, Howard Bennett rid himself of sleep apnea, leg edema, high blood pressure, high cholesterol, and bad back problems. All this in only 26 months!

way was about as far as I could go. But I kept trying. After about a week, I made it to the end of the block. And by the end of the following week, I made it all the way around the block.

"It took me about five weeks to build up to a mile. Then I started increasing my pace. After about nine months, I was walking an hour a day—covering about 3½ to 4 miles. In the past 20 months, I've walked 2,778 miles."

A New Life

"I've lost 340 pounds, but I've never gained any back. And my waistline has dropped from 78 inches to 34!

"As for my diet, I can eat practically as much as I want now as long as I still limit my fats. My favorite snacking food is popcorn cakes—and there's no fat in them.

"My health has improved dramatically. I used to take over $200 worth of medicine every month just for my high blood pressure and diabetes. And I haven't had to for almost 1½ years now. My blood pressure is normal—120/87—and my diabetes is gone. My cholesterol is very low—146. When I went to the doctor a few months ago, he said, 'You really don't need to lose any more. You're perfectly fine right where you are.'

"It's such a drastic change. Now there's nothing that really limits me. I still have to be careful lifting things because of my back. But I can go places—I can go to the movies now. I can go to restaurants and sit in a regular booth—and the table's way away from my belly. I can get behind the wheel of my car. It's like being reborn!

"Recently, I flew to Florida for my 30-year class reunion. My old classmates barely recognized me. I had been heavy all through school, and they expected me to be heavy now. And there I was, a normal weight. They even named me 'Most Changed for the Better.'

"No wonder. I haven't weighed this little since I left grammar school."

CHAPTER

8

ANSWERS TO DIETERS' MOST COMMON QUESTIONS

A lot of sensible would-be weight losers stumble along the way because they have unanswered questions about the changes they're being asked to make. After all, if you don't know why it's important to cut fat intake, or exactly the best way to do it, how good are your chances for success? And if you're not fully armed with the facts, what are your chances of fending off the false promise of quick weight-loss schemes?

To help, here is a compilation of the most troublesome questions that weight-control specialists are asked most often. The answers may be able to quench your curiosity, send some myths up in smoke, and give you the kind of down-to-earth helpful tips that can put the punch back in your weight-loss program.

Q Diets always seem to recommend drinking eight glasses of water a day. Can this really have an effect on weight loss?

A Yes, but not for the reasons you may think. It's not because water "flushes toxins out of your system" or "fills you up." The real reason is that water can kill certain cravings.

Many people habitually misinterpret cravings for fluid as food cravings. The result: They eat to satisfy their thirst.

The key to quenching such cravings with water lies not so much in the quantity you drink as in how frequently you drink it. Small amounts (3 to 4 ounces) sipped frequently work better than 8 ounces downed like medicine.

The next time you experience what you think is a food craving, try sipping a small cup of water. If it's fluid your body really hungers for, you should be able to avert the craving and forget you even wanted a bite to eat.

But note: Water means water, not coffee, tea, diet soda, fruit juice, or any other fluid. The goal is to satisfy thirst, not stimulate your taste buds.

Q Can a high-protein diet help me retain lean muscle while losing fat?

A A moderate amount of protein is necessary to maintain muscle mass while losing weight. You can easily meet your protein needs, however, on a carefully designed low-fat, high-carbohydrate diet. For most people, this is the safest, most effective diet for long-term weight control.

It appears that a daily intake of at least 65 grams of protein is needed to reduce loss of muscle tissue while dieting. By eating small portions of lean meat and low-fat or nonfat dairy products, along with generous amounts of grains, vegetables and legumes, you can easily satisfy your protein requirements—and your appetite!

Try to get two-thirds of your protein from vegetable sources like beans, grains, and soy products. Even though vegetable sources are significantly lower in protein than animal sources, they are high in fiber and generally lower in fat.

Here are a few figures for high-protein foods that may help you plan: There are about 24 grams of protein in 3 ounces of cooked lean meat, fish, or fowl; 8 grams in an 8-ounce glass of low-fat milk; 18 grams in a 4-ounce serving of tofu; about 8 grams in ½ cup of legumes. Most other cooked vegetables have about 2 grams per ½ cup. Keep in mind, too, that exercise, especially resistance training with light weights, can help build and maintain your muscle mass while burning fat.

Q Is it harder to lose weight as you get older?

A Actually, not much. Metabolism (the rate at which we burn calories) changes only 1 to 2 percent per decade. What does change for most of us is lifestyle. The older we get, the more efficient we become at conserving energy—like finding parking spots nearer the store. It only takes 1 percent here, 2 percent there, to add up to sizable savings. As our muscle mass declines with disuse, the percentage of body fat increases. Burning 100 fewer calories per day (the amount used in about 20 minutes of housecleaning, gardening or brisk walking) can mean gaining 10 pounds in a year.

If you want to keep your weight stable, the solution is to keep moving. It takes approximately 200 minutes of purposeful movement, like housecleaning or climbing steps, per week to beat the system.

Q What is cellulite, and is there anything I can do to get rid of it?

A That dimply, orange-peel look of the skin around the hips, buttocks, and thighs, which has been dubbed "cellulite," is nothing more than a buildup of fat cells. Women are more susceptible than men because they're genetically determined to carry more fat in those areas. Men also have a thicker network of fibrous connective tissue in the skin, which helps it maintain a more uniform tone.

While fat distribution is primarily genetic, weight gain or lack of physical fitness can push a propensity into a reality. Dropping excess pounds and stepping up aerobic activity are the best solutions for those who are overweight. Normal-weight women who are troubled by this condition may find that regular exercise (both aerobic and resistance training) will help by reducing their overall body fat and improving muscle tone.

Also note that no cream, massage, or any other type of exterior manipulation has been proved to exert the slightest change on cellulite.

Q How can I enhance the resiliency of my skin while I lose weight?

A There are four ways to accomplish this: (1) Lose slowly. Recommendations for weight-loss pace have recently been reduced: ½ to 1 pound per week is best; (2) Keep it off. (Yo-yo-ing overtaxes skin elasticity); (3) Maintain good protein levels. (Skin needs protein as much as muscle does); (4) Get plenty of exercise. Resistance types like light weight training are best.

Q How can I suppress my craving for chocolate?

A Real food cravings/addictions (not lack of water) are hard to extinguish. It takes commitment and willpower. To succeed, you must go on the wagon for 12 weeks. That's about the length of time it seems to take for a person to adjust successfully to new habits.

Q Why can't I seem to eat only one potato chip?

A Because it's not a serving size. While there's no such thing as a one-size-fits-all serving, a single chip is unlikely to meet anyone's idea of satisfaction.

In addition, salt is one of those flavors that jolt the taste buds and set them clamoring for more: "I like that! Do it again!" (Sweet, bitter, and sour are other tastes that can overexcite the mouth.) So try to snack on foods low in fat, sodium, and sugar, and high in fiber, such as air-popped popcorn or fruit.

Q Why does weight loss go faster at the start of a diet, then slow down?

A Because you're losing different types of body weight at each stage. During the initial stages of caloric restriction, you lose fat, muscle, and water. After about two weeks, loss of muscle and water slows. Then somewhere between weeks three and five, you actually start to regain the muscle and water weight you originally lost. (That's the dreaded "plateau.") You may even gain weight, since muscle (which you're gaining) weighs more than fat (which you're losing). But stick with it: As long as you're faithful to your diet and exercise, you should still lose body fat.

Minimizing loss of muscle is a big reason why slow weight loss is recommended. Those who lose more than ½ to 1 pound a week simply lose a greater proportion of muscle and water, to be inevitably regained later.

To prevent diet burnout (discouragement caused by a plateau), stop using the scale to monitor your progress. Instead use the "sum of circumferences" (take your measurements and add them up). Decreasing inches reflect loss of body fat better than decreasing pounds.

Experts also recommend that once dieters have lost 10 percent of their total body weight, they take a break and give their body time to adjust. It seems that the body or brain (we aren't yet sure which regulates this) only wants to lose 5 to 10 percent at one time. After a 12-week maintenance period, you'll be ready—body and mind—to take off another 10 percent, if that's appropriate for you.

Q I've heard that if you cut calories too much, you "downshift" your metabolism. How much is too much?

A In general, your body doesn't want to cut back more than 500 calories a day, or 1 pound a week. Any time you go beyond that, you shock the system. Your body kicks into the classical stress response as it prepares for what it perceives to be a famine. Exaggerated adrenaline production and other stress reactions can make you feel shaky, queasy, and light-headed. If you feel like this, you know you've cut back too far.

Q Why is it that every time I go on a diet it gets harder and harder for me to take the weight off?

A Don't take off weight you can't keep off! Yo-yo dieting is not only tough on your health in general, it also makes further weight loss more difficult. Here's why: The enzyme responsible for storing fat (called lipoprotein lipase, or LPL), found on the surface of fat tissue, has a memory. The LPL of the first-time dieter is ignorant. When it stops getting the amount of fat it's used to, it takes a while to realize it needs to produce more enzyme to attract (and store) more fat. The more often a person goes on and off diets, the more he's training his LPL to produce enzyme and store fat more quickly and efficiently.

The solution is to lose slowly and exercise. Don't fall prey to weight-loss schemes that promise speed. They don't work. The biggest virtue for a dieter is patience.

Q How long after an aerobic workout do I continue to burn calories at a higher rate?

A It depends. The longer and more intense the workout, the longer and greater the afterburn. A 30-minute brisk walk should keep your metabolism revved up for about 4 extra hours. While that's certainly not enough to allow you a triple-fudge sundae, don't underestimate the importance of small gains. A workout also boosts metabolism by increasing muscle mass, and muscle burns more calories than fat—even at rest.

Q I have no problem taking weight off. My problem is keeping it off. What am I doing wrong?

A It can't be repeated often enough: One secret to keeping weight off is an aerobic fitness program. You've got to make walking or other aerobic activity an integral part of your lifestyle. Otherwise, you'll almost certainly put the weight back on.

Too many people rely strictly on diets to lose weight. At ten weeks of dieting there's a 95 percent quit rate. It's like hitting a wall. If you haven't built up a pretty good exercise program by then, your weight-loss efforts are doomed. By burning calories and body fat (which begins to "melt" after the first 20 minutes of an aerobic workout), regular exercise allows you to control your weight while eating enough to satisfy your hunger.

Q Is exercise an appetite suppressant?

A Yes, up to a point. For many people, a walk of 30 to 40 minutes at least every other day can help put the lid on a ravenous appetite. But don't overdo it; vigorous exercise can sometime stimulate your appetite. Muscle aches, exhaustion, or feeling excessively hungry are signs you need to back off.

Q Are appetite-suppressant pills considered safe?

A Used as directed, yes. But they are not a substitute for a sensible weight-loss program, which includes a low-fat, high-carbohydrate diet, moderate exercise, and behavior modification. Appetite suppressants may have a valid place in a physician-supervised weight-loss program, but only after all other means have failed and only when used in addition to other sound weight-loss principles.

Q Are there foods that should be avoided because they stimulate the appetite?

A Not exactly, but some foods can make dieting more difficult. Some highly caloric drinks add empty calories without satisfying the craving for food. High-fructose corn syrup, which is found in many sodas, and alcohol both have this effect. The body simply does not perceive these liquids as satisfying, so after drinking them, the urge to eat remains.

Fat poses a similar problem. It could be called a craving enhancer because it always leaves you wanting more.

Q Does weight loss really make gallstone attacks more likely?

A Rapid weight loss increases the chance of developing gallstones by 10 to 100 times. On the other hand, obesity also raises the risk significantly—the risk of gallstones from obesity rises the heavier you get, up to 50 times the risk of a person of normal weight. What's a person to do? Slow but steady wins this race, reducing the chance of gallstones to that of the normal population. Also important: Once you've lost those pounds, keep them off. Rapid weight loss and gain and binge eating increase risk of gallstones.

Q Is it true that certain foods can cancel calories from other foods?

A This concept of special foods having "negative caloric action" is hogwash. There are no magical foods that cancel other calories you consume, despite the myth that surrounds grapefruit.

But there are foods that allow a person to fill up before consuming too many calories. A diet that emphasizes protein and complex carbohydrates allows you to feel satiated and still end up with a negative caloric intake after you account for expenditure through exercise.

The problem with fat calories is that they're devilishly easy to overconsume because they taste so darn good. Also, because of lipoprotein lipase, fat calories are more easily stored than protein or carbohydrates. Often they're stored so fast that you don't even get the chance to burn them, leaving you hungry sooner and more apt to eat.

Q What role should fiber supplements play in a safe and effective weight-loss plan?

A A supplemental one. The recommended intake for dietary fiber is 20 to 35 grams per day. Most Americans get only between 10 and 15 grams. Somehow, people need to get a high-fiber kicker in there. If you've exhausted your ability to consume fiber from foods, you may want to take a supplement to help you reach your quota. As long as the majority of your intake comes from natural sources (at least 15 grams), then getting another 10 grams from supplements can be a real boost. The recommended types of fiber supplements are powdered or flaky (such as psyllium and bran) rather than fiber pills, which can expand and cause medical problems.

Q Every month I have PMS, and one of my symptoms is carbohydrate cravings. Is there anything that can help me beat the PMS cravings and stay on my diet?

A Scientists do not yet fully understand what causes the collection of symptoms known as Premenstrual Syndrome (PMS). Judith Wurtman, Ph.D., a research scientist in the Department of Brain and Cognitive Sciences at the Massachusetts Institute of Technology and author of *Managing Your Mind and Mood through Food*, explains that when you are dieting you often reduce your intake of carbohydrates, and this may make your premenstrual cravings even worse. She recommends that you eat some carbohydrates daily and perhaps eat increased amounts during the week before your period. "Women with PMS food cravings should not expect to lose weight steadily throughout the month. They should be content if they can lose weight three weeks out of every four," says Dr. Wurtman.

Q I have recently lost a lot of weight, and as a result, the skin on my neck under my chin is loose and flabby. My question is: Are there any exercises you can advise to tighten this skin without surgery?

A Yes, we came up with one. But first, others should know that this problem can be avoided entirely if you do a little strength training during your weight-loss period.

Anyone who's losing weight should also do strength training (push-ups, chin-ups, or light work with dumbbells and/or strength machines) 20 minutes a day three times a week to prevent muscle loss from occurring. That's what happened in this particular case—muscle was lost with all that weight.

Now here's your exercise. You need to work your platysma muscle, which you do anytime you make a funny face or when you grimace. Push out your lower jaw—really push out those bottom teeth as far as you can, and you should feel it tightening up those muscles under your chin.

Any facial expression will do that to some degree, but this one really pulls that muscle in tight. Hold it for 10 seconds and start by doing ten of those twice a day. Build up gradually, increasing the number of times you do it and the number of times a day, and you should see some real improvement.

Q As part of my weight-loss regimen, I have been exercising daily. Lately, my wife complains that I'm not the man I used to be. Could my exercise program be cooling my sex drive?

A Several scientists have looked into the matter. They say that heavy training may drain the male anatomy of some of its sex-inspiring hormones.

Researchers from the University of Alberta found testosterone levels in 31 male runners averaging 40 miles a week to be a good 30 percent lower than the levels in 18 nonrunners. The Canadian scientists speculate that the stress of rigorous training mimics times in our prehistoric past when sex would have been a bad idea—during extended hunts, for example, or difficult migrations. The cavemen who gave into their sexual desire during the mastodon hunt may have gone hungry.

Exactly how soon overtraining takes its toll on the sex drive and how long the negative effects last remain a mystery. However, Rudolph Dressendorfer, Ph.D., director of the human performance lab at New Mexico Highlands University, who co-directed a similar study a few years ago, says that 15 to 60 minutes of vigorous exercise three to five days a week should not alter testosterone levels or sex drive.

Q I love pizza. I eat it at least once, often twice, a week. Bad news?

A Not necessarily. Pizza is fattening only if you eat too much of it. How much is too much? It depends. One slice with pepperoni and sausage packs about 275 calories, but a slice with mushrooms and peppers can clock in at less than 120 calories.

One thing is a given: The bigger the pie you buy, the more pizza you'll eat. Forget about bringing home enough to have leftovers for breakfast; get the small size or order by the slice.

Q I'm an allergy sufferer—upper respiratory, hay fever, itchy eyes and throat. After a few doses of my prescription allergy medication, my appetite seems to increase in leaps and bounds. Could my allergy medicine be sabotaging my weight-loss efforts?

A Your hunger could be caused by a "rebound effect" due to a drug called phenylpropanolamine, which may be in the antihistamine/decongestant medications you are taking. That's also the same active ingredient that is in diet pills. The problem is, when you go off the over-the-counter drugs or diet pills, you may experience an increase in hunger.

Frank Greenway, M.D., a professor of medicine at the University of California, Los Angeles, explains this rebound effect: "Once you go off these drugs, the body will do what it needs to get back to its original weight level. Each individual has a weight that the body strives to maintain, called the body set point. Your increased appetite may be your body trying to adjust itself."

While you are on these appetite-suppressing medications, maintain your diet. Don't stop eating. If you're not sure which medications contain phenylpropanolamine, check the labels.

Q Why do I tend to eat more at big family gatherings?

A Gluttony loves company. The more mouths at the dinner table, the more you can count on eating. At least, that's what researchers found when they checked diet records and eating habits of about 80 average eaters. They looked at many factors—including where people ate, what type of meal they ate, and whether they had eaten beforehand. But the factor that had the most influence on the amount a person packed away was the number of people he or she ate with. Put simply, more mouths meant more mouthfuls.

"The biggest leap in calories came when people went from eating alone to eating with one other person," says John M. de Castro, Ph.D., associate professor of psychology at Georgia State University. "The amount of food eaten went up nearly 50 percent." But the increase didn't stop there. The extra calories continued to build as more people joined the meal.

This doesn't mean you have to skip dinner with your spouse because you're battling the bulge. But you can be mindful of the mob, and realize eating in a group poses more challenges than simply remembering people's names. If you know you're going to be having dinner with a crowd, for example, you can plan ahead by eating a leaner lunch. If you're dining out, stick to lower-fat items on the menu—salad with a squeeze of fresh lemon (instead of dressing), broiled fish or chicken, steamed vegetables, and unbuttered bread. And to help keep wandering hands from fulfilling your cravings, keep them busy by holding onto a glass of water or low-calorie soda.

The chief authority for this chapter was George L. Blackburn, M.D., Ph.D., associate professor of surgery at Harvard Medical School and chief of the Nutrition/Metabolism Laboratory with the Cancer Research Institute at New England Deaconess Hospital, Boston. Other consultants included Phil Dunphy, physical therapist, exercise physiologist, and former owner of Health through Exercise and Rehabilitation (HEAR); Dr. Judith Wurtman; Dr. Rudolph Dressendorfer; Dr. Frank Greenway; and Dr. John de Castro.

THE DIET DETECTIVE: A CRITICAL LOOK AT WEIGHT-LOSS AIDS AND TECHNOLOGY

With all the diet products and practices on the market today, it can be very hard to tell which ones will make you lose weight and which ones will make you lose money. Dieters can be suckers when it comes to easy weight-loss promises.

This chapter is designed to help you decipher the truth about some of the products and services available to you. It should dispel a few myths and help you trim the "fat" from the facts.

Flab-Fighting Fiction

"I can't tell you what's in the pill because they don't tell us the ingredients; all we're supposed to say is that it is derived from 100 percent natural plant sources and contains no drugs or stimulants," says an employee for one diet pill that claims its $19.95-per-bottle pills will rid you of so-called cellulite in 30 days. (It's one of the cheapest cellulite-removing products on the market.) "But I know that it's completely safe."

Others hope to remove a hefty amount of your paycheck along with your flab. For nearly $500, a mail-order firm offers a device that claims to melt fat (while building muscle) by means of electrical stimulation. "The stimulation causes the muscles to flex and relax, which tones the body," says the saleswoman. "If you do it for 15 minutes a day, you'll get rid of your cellulite in no time, while building your muscle as if you were lifting weights."

The device, she claims, "works on all fat, but it works *best* on cellulite. And I assure you, it's totally safe." (No doubt, since it's powered by a 9-volt battery, like that found in a transistor radio.)

A cheaper and equally effective—and less dangerous—alternative is your morning cup of brew. "Even if you wore one of those devices all day, it wouldn't kick up your metabolism any higher than a cup of coffee does," says physiologist William Stauber, Ph.D., of West Virginia University, an expert in neuromuscular electrical stimulation. "In principle, this device would build muscle if the charge were strong enough, but you couldn't do it without close medical supervision."

Even liposuction, a surgical procedure costing anywhere from $2,000 to $5,000, in which fat is sucked out from well under the skin, may not help to remove dimpled fat. In fact, says Richard Dolsky, M.D., a Philadelphia plastic surgeon who was one of the first to teach the procedure in the United States, "it may make it worse. So-called cellulite is a skin condition, and it's not one that any reputable plastic surgeon can claim to cure permanently. Surgeons who do liposuction are very careful not to get near the skin. The fat that is removed is well below it."

While help for dimpled thighs and sagging butts may not be in the advertisements in the back of magazines, there is hope: Like other problems related to fat, some "cellulite," if not most, can be lost through diet and exercise.

"You've got to burn the excess fat," says personal fitness trainer Stu Mittleman. "That means exercising aerobically—walking, jogging, swimming, or biking—at a pace moderate enough that you can sustain it for a fairly long time, like half an hour. Burning fat is not the same as burning calories. You have to reach a heart rate of about 60 percent of your maximum and keep it there for at least 20 minutes before you start burning fat."

Another way to minimize dimpled fat is to build and tone the muscles under the fat layer. "Exercise doesn't convert fat to muscle, but firm, toned muscles may help smooth out the skin and reduce the appearance of cellulite," adds Mittleman. Besides exercising, you should eat a diet that gets no more than 30 percent of its calories from fat—most of which should be unsaturated or monounsaturated fats, like those found in vegetables and fish.

"It may make some women feel better to say 'I have

a cellulite problem,' when really what they should be saying is 'I have a fat butt,' " says Maria Simonson, Ph.D., Sc.D., director of the Health, Weight, and Stress Program at Johns Hopkins Medical Institutions in Baltimore. "But if you're not overweight, and if you're in good shape, you don't have cellulite."

Subliminal Weight-Loss Tapes— Electronic Snake Oil

You may have heard of "subliminal" audiocassette tapes that promise to reshape your mind and body.

"They are a form of health fraud," says Timothy Moore, Ph.D., former chairman of the Psychology Department at Glendon College, York University in Toronto. "While subliminal perception is a respectable area of investigation in clinical psychology, these tapes are another example of a little truth carried to extremes. It's just preposterous for the people who sell these things to claim that they can change your whole life."

Anthony Greenwald, Ph.D., professor of psychology at the University of Washington, Seattle, is inclined to agree. "After a series of experiments under actual use conditions—that is, people taking these things home and using them just like the directions say you should—my colleagues, Dr. Anthony Pratkanis and Eric Spangenberg, and I are dubious that these tapes have any effect at all subliminally."

Catalogs promising "effortless self-improvement"—be it weight loss, increased self-confidence, or a better golf score—abound. The tapes they're pushing claim to have "powerful subliminal messages" embedded in sound tracks of ocean waves, New Age or Baroque music, and other monotonous, albeit relaxing, noises. The catalogs maintain that even though our ears can't hear the cascade of messages stuck subliminally under the waves, our sub-conscious not only hears but also can be shaped by it.

Subliminal Perception Is Real, but . . .

All the psychologists interviewed by *Prevention* agreed that most people *do* have subliminal perception, which essentially means we can respond to outside signals, images, or messages without being consciously aware of them, or aware that we are responding. Some controlled scientific studies have demonstrated an apparent impact of subliminal *visual* signals. But not one repeatable study has shown that allegedly "subliminal" audio signals have any impact on behavior—for one simple reason. Our ears are *physically incapable* of distinguishing words below the level of hearing. "Subliminal sound" is a contradiction in terms—a sound that is imperceptible is not a sound.

Consider this: If you were in the Louvre when the lights went out, you couldn't *see* the Mona Lisa, but it would still be hanging there. Raising or lowering sound beyond certain levels is akin to "turning out the lights" on your ears. The sound may still be there, but if it doesn't stimulate your brain, there's no information to process. And no information means no impact.

"It is possible to show a picture, word, or phrase so quickly that people will say they haven't seen it, even when they have," says Dr. Moore. "Some controlled studies have shown that some visual stimuli do have a measurable influence on behavior, although none of these has anything to do with clinical change.

"The key difference between visual and audible signals, though, is that although you can sharply reduce the amount of time it's visible, people still see that picture," he explains. "Say, for example, you show slides that say 'Eat less' or 'Don't smoke'. No matter how fast they appear and disappear, the message doesn't change.

"But with sound, speeding up the message, which is what some of these tapes claim to do, changes the stimulus, the message. We're dealing with the physics of speech. If you speed up the spoken message, you change the sound waves, and you don't have 'Eat less' or 'Don't smoke' anymore."

As a matter of fact, says Dr. Moore, when you can hear them, the speeded-up words sound like ripping cloth.

A Double Rip-Off: Sometimes No Message at All

Not only is the message changed on some of these tapes, sometimes it's not there at all, says another Canadian researcher, Philip Merikle, Ph.D., of the University of Waterloo.

Dr. Merikle took several "subliminal" tapes and put them through a spectrographic analysis. The sonic spectrograph "hears" sounds within the ability of the human ear, regardless of how speeded-up, high-pitched, or faint. Then it indicates the frequencies of those sounds by making lines on paper. So, no matter how altered, if spoken suggestions were embedded in the soundtrack of the tapes, they would show up.

The result? "The spectrographic analyses suggest that these subliminal cassettes do not contain any embedded messages," writes Dr. Merikle in *Psychology and Marketing.* In other words, there's nothing on some of them except the sounds of the ocean or the New Wave music or the whatever.

So there's a double rip-off—some tape manufacturers don't even go to the trouble of putting a "subliminal" track, which won't accomplish anything even if it is there, on their products.

But *Affirmations* Can Influence You

After all this, is anything to be said in favor of subliminal self-improvement tapes?

Yes, there is. Even the subliminals, say our experts, may have a "placebo" effect. That is, the user expects it to work, so it does. But Dr. Moore and Dr. Greenwald emphasize that such an effect is fickle and temporary. "The therapeutic effect is just not there," says Dr. Moore. "There might be a way to reach the subconscious mind, but subliminal audiotapes are not it."

Tapes full of affirmations that you can *hear*, however, such as "I can eat less," or "I like to exercise" can really be an effective part of therapy, says psychologist Irene Vogel, Ph.D., who uses them in her Washington, D.C.–area practice. "I use them for some of my clients who need to change their attitudes and perceptions about certain things."

But even those tapes *alone* aren't going to accomplish anything, especially for people who have psychological barriers to overcome before they can lose weight, says Dr. Vogel.

"For example, a woman who uses her fat for protection—from unwanted sexual attention, from being involved in things, or whatever—will self-sabotage any success she may have at dieting. A tape isn't going to overcome that. And that's where I see a real problem with these tapes, at least for some people. They're going to turn to them, when really they should be seeking professional help."

Dr. Vogel is also beginning to explore the use of videotapes with subliminal messages on them. "I've asked several clients to watch them in the waiting room before they start their sessions. They know they are getting subliminal messages, and what those messages are, so right now this is not controlled research in any sense. But my clients, some of whom are trying to lose weight or quit smoking, and others who are working on issues of confidence and goal setting, are quite enthusiastic."

As Dr. Moore and others pointed out, there is some evidence that visual subliminal messages can have an impact. So subliminal self-help videotapes may have effects that the audiotapes most certainly do not.

The Perils and Pitfalls of Liquid Fasting Diets
By Molly O'Neill
of the New York Times

It has been almost two years since Oprah Winfrey rapidly dropped 67 pounds on a liquid formula diet and contributed to a nationwide renaissance of the weight-loss method. And nearly a million Americans are trying to establish normal eating habits after the fast, health professionals estimate.

Some people develop a fear of food and become dependent on formula diets. Others binge and suffer humiliating weight gains. Few maintain their lower weights. A five-year study by Dr. Thomas Wadden of the University of Pennsylvania showed that 98 percent of all dieters regain their weight within five years. The liquid diet industry, the medical profession, entrepreneurs, major pharmaceutical companies, and individual dieters are all hungry for a sliver of success. But interviews over two months with 31 patients after fasting—and recent medical studies—suggest that the nature of the formula diets could lead to psychological and physiological burdens that limit the diets' long-term effectiveness.

Lose 100 Pounds, Regain 120

"Last year, everybody knew somebody who'd lost 100 pounds on a fast," says Barry Adler, president of Diet Fast, a formula diet program. "Now, everybody knows somebody who lost 100 pounds and gained back 120."

Across the country, dozens of obesity specialists have noticed an increase in patients on the fast-and-binge roller coaster.

At a conference of the American Federation of the American Societies for Experimental Biology (FASEB) in Washington, D.C., Dr. Adam Drewnowski, director of human nutrition at the University of Michigan, presented findings that yo-yo dieting—cycles of rapid weight loss and gain frequently associated with liquid formula diets—creates a craving for calorie-dense mixtures of sugar and fat.

Dr. Theodore VanItallie, a consultant of the United Weight Control Corporation, a formula weight-loss program based in Englewood Cliffs, New Jersey, has been in the vanguard of obesity study for 27 years. He has concluded that rapid weight loss can be sustained only by long-term psychological support and nutritional education.

The Promise

By 1988, according to MarketData Enterprises, a research group in Lynbrook, New York, diet clinics were a $10-billion-a-year industry, and hospital-sponsored programs generated $5.5 billion more. Liquid formula diets are now the fastest-growing segment of the country's weight-loss industry, MarketData has reported.

In the House of Representatives, the Small Business Subcommittee on Regulation, Business Opportunities, and Energy plans major hearings. "We are very concerned about the false promises, lack of efficacy, high cost, and astounding failure rate of liquid diets," says the subcommittee chairman, Representative Ron Wyden (D-Oregon).

His concern is shared in the field itself. William Rush, a senior vice-president of Optifast programs, said the diets "are only appropriate for severely obese patients."

Formula diet advertising typically invokes "clinical studies" and offers happy statistics. To date, none are based on long-term, independent studies.

"In no other field of medicine can people who know so little claim to do so much," says Dr. VanItallie.

The Realities

"A drug addict stands a better chance of recovery than a dieter," says Dr. Phillip M. Sinaikin, director of the adult substance-abuse treatment program at Fair Oaks Hospital in Summit, New Jersey. In his book *After the Fast,* Dr. Sinaikin outlines a nine-week plan for steady, rapid weight loss. He advocates nutritional education, behavior modification, and exercise.

Many obesity experts say such a coolly measured prescription is doomed. "If these patients were capable of being rational about food, they wouldn't have the problem in the first place," said Dr. Stephen Gullo, a Manhattan obesity expert. "Abstaining from food doesn't teach people how to live with food."

Abstinence may even activate the physiological and psychological demons that haunt fasters like the shadows of their former selves. At the FASEB meeting, Dr. Drenowski presented evidence that repeated crash diets may change food preferences. Following up animal studies done at Yale, he found that humans who dieted often and severely developed cravings for fat and sugar.

Of 31 formula diet patients interviewed over two months, 23 said their food preferences changed during the fast. To many, the unfamiliar urges became uncontrollable and ultimately humiliating. Most of the dieters asked to remain anonymous.

Few Successes, Many Rebounds

Jay, a 44-year-old real estate developer in Los Angeles, has been nearly 200 pounds overweight most of his adult life. In 1981, he undertook a medically monitored formula diet for ten months and two days, and lost 194 pounds.

"I felt great, but I had these fantasies of eating steak," he said. "I'd never been much of a meat eater, but suddenly I had these nonstop steak fantasies." He said he gained the weight back in 12 months, lost it again, then regained 220 pounds. He plans to begin the liquid diet again.

Many people concede, after their fasting period, that they have battled intense psychological pressure. "I see it all the time," says Dr. Gullo. "These patients know that they've only learned not to eat. Why wouldn't they be terrified to eat again?" Jacques, 47, a Manhattan lawyer, religiously took a liquid formula diet for several months and lost 143 pounds. Then he started dreaming of food. "Christmas night I woke my wife up because I was sweating over David's Cookies," he says.

One Friday, Jacques closed his office door, drew up an itinerary, and hired a car and driver for the next day. From noon to 7:30 P.M. that Saturday, he sat in the back seat eating.

His calm "I-deserve-this" air overshadowed the bizarre 22-stop adventure. Wrappers and carry-out food containers cluttered the car. About 7,000 calories later, Jacques told a reporter, "I am going back on formula tomorrow."

He had gained 21 pounds in 13 days.

Like many fasters, he had been in control of not eating. He was also an impeccably organized master of his binges. It is the middle ground between the two extremes that confounds him and many other people after the fast.

Don't Crash Diet!
Fasting Triggers Unbearable
Cravings for Fats and Sweets

Shortly after his presentation at the FASEB conference mentioned in the previous section, *Prevention* asked Dr. Adam Drewnowski's opinion on fasting for weight loss, and whether he thought fasters were setting themselves up for weight-loss failure.

"In the study I presented," he says, "We gave a large number of obese people samples of cake-frosting-like mixtures that ranged up to 35 percent fat and 70 percent sucrose. We confirmed something that had already been found in animal tests: People with a history of losing weight and gaining it back, over and over—yo-yo dieting, in other words—had definite preferences for the sweetest, fattiest foods in our sample. It seems that crash dieting, when people are being very strict with themselves, triggers these cravings for the highest-calorie foods.

"That seems to be one problem with fasts, which are sort of the ultimate crash diets. They can set up these nearly unbearable cravings for foods that put the weight back on very fast. Some people go off a fast and just binge on very calorie-dense foods.

"I'm not against fasting per se. Under the right medical supervision, properly chosen patients can safely lose weight that they wouldn't otherwise. What is very dangerous is unsupervised, self-selected fasting.

"I think that many of the people who resort to fasting, who look on it as their 'last chance,' are intractably obese; that is, their genetic makeup is such that they are fighting an impossible battle. They can fast and lose the weight, but when they start eating again, they will gain it all back.

"That's why an examination by a qualified doctor is so important. An expert can determine if a fast really is the best way for someone to attempt to lose weight and set a realistic goal for them.

"There are some good, well-supervised medical fasting programs, such as Optifast. They have very strict criteria, not only for selecting patients but also for the doctors who administer the therapy. They also try to teach people how to eat when they go back to solid food again. But most of the commercial programs that are available in shopping centers have no professional supervision—no doctors, no nurses, no registered dietitians. They take anybody, regardless of their health, without insisting they have a medical checkup first.

"No one should attempt to diet—let alone fast—without a doctor's help."

Rotation Diets Don't Work

Remember the Rotation Diet? That was where you ate a very-low-calorie diet for a few days, then a moderately low one, then a near-normal one, then back to the very low, and so on. The idea was that this would keep your metabolism (and thus your calorie-burning) from slowing down. Also, it was supposed to be easier to stick with, since you knew the deprivation periods would be brief.

It seemed like a good idea, but dieting doesn't work that way. Studies in Tennessee and California that tried various combinations of alternating food intakes, with and without exercise, all came to the conclusion that the Rotation Diet has no effect on resting metabolic rate and is no better than steady, moderate calorie restriction at reducing weight.

Will the 1990s Bring Back Cyclamates?

Cyclamates, banned in 1970 after a cancer scare, may make a comeback in the 1990s, predicts Patricia McLaughlin, Ph.D., consumer safety officer at the Food and Drug Administration (FDA). This is good news for calorie counters, since this calorie-free sweetener leaves no annoying aftertaste as does saccharin, and it doesn't lose its sweetness when heated, as does aspartame.

"The ban was based on the findings of one study, which was criticized from the start," says Dr. McLaughlin. "In 1984, the FDA's Cancer Assessment Committee reviewed a lot of later studies and agreed that the cancer fears were groundless."

Abbott Laboratories, the manufacturer, petitioned the FDA to lift the ban. But although the FDA cleared the cancer charges, they still had some questions about cyclamates' safety. Some studies have shown that the sweetener causes testicular atrophy and embryo poisoning in rats.

The FDA will review data on the sweetener's role, if any, in temporary high blood pressure in some people. The next step for the agency would be an overall safety assessment of the substance, Dr. McLaughlin says. "The FDA will move very slowly on this. Artificial sweeteners are used by millions of people, so we have to be as sure as we can that cyclamates are safe."

Diet Sodas May Help Tame Your Sweet Tooth

Diet soda can reduce the urge for eating sweets when consumed regularly, suggests a study by M. G. Tordoff, Ph.D., of the Monell Chemical Senses Center in Philadelphia. Although artificial sweeteners provide no nutritional value, Dr. Tordoff found that they can be a beneficial dieting tool: When test subjects drank five cups (3.3 cans) of diet soda a day for three weeks, they ate fewer sweets, enabling them to reduce caloric intake. When they consumed the same amount of regular soda, however, it had no effect on their eating habits.

And here's additional good news for people with a sweet tooth. A recent study found no evidence of a link between artificial sweeteners (often used in diet soda) and bladder cancer, as some scientists had suspected. Investigators looked for cancer cells in the autopsied bladders of 149 people who had answered questionnaires about artificial sweetener use. People with bladder cancer were no more likely to have used saccharin, cyclamates, or aspartame than people without bladder cancer, say the researchers at the Veterans Administration Medical Center in East Orange, New Jersey.

Fake Fats: Are the Benefits Real?

If your quest for good nutrition sometimes leaves you craving ice cream, fries, or double dollops of sour cream, you've probably been intrigued by recent reports of synthetic fat that promises to make such foods more healthful. Like sugar substitutes, phony fat is destined to take a prominent place in the American diet. But is it really a boon to health and fitness? Is it even safe?

Olestra

Procter and Gamble stumbled upon Olestra nearly 20 years ago while trying to formulate a source of nourishment for premature infants. By chemically binding a sugar to the fatty acids in vegetable oil, they discovered a compound called sucrose polyester that has the look, taste, feel, and satiety value of real fat. But because sucrose polyester cannot be broken down by digestive enzymes, it passes through the body without contributing calories.

By replacing much of the high-calorie fat in shortening, cooking oil, margarine, salad dressings, ice cream, baked goods, snack chips, and deep-fried foods, Olestra could make life easier for the weight-conscious. And there might be health benefits for everyone. If early studies prove correct, Olestra could be a potent cholesterol reducer that works by replacing some of the saturated fat in our diet and by picking up excess cholesterol in the intestines as it passes through. Better yet, sucrose polyester seems to lower only LDL (bad) cholesterol without affecting the HDL (good) variety.

If Olestra seems too good to be true, it just might be. Because sucrose polyester acts like fat, it mixes with fat-soluble vitamins such as A and E and removes them from the body. While this problem can probably be solved by fortifying Olestra with vitamins, there are more serious issues. In Procter and Gamble's initial safety study, the substance caused pituitary tumors, leukemia, abnormal liver changes, early mortality, and birth defects in rats. Some findings improved in a subsequent test, but the pituitary and liver problems persisted.

Because sucrose polyester is not absorbed by the body (implying that it should be safe), the FDA exempted

Procter and Gamble from testing a second rodent species, something normally required of food additives that may be consumed in large amounts. But the Center for Science in the Public Interest (CSPI) petitioned the company for additional testing, and it agreed to perform a lifetime study of mice, putting FDA approval of Olestra at least two years away.

While Procter and Gamble literature promotes the safety of Olestra on the grounds that it is an all-natural substance made from sugar and vegetable oil, CSPI scientist Lisa Leffert points out that these substances have been chemically changed to produce "a new molecule that is totally foreign to the body." Because a chemical change can transform a harmless substance into a toxic one, serious questions about Olestra's safety remain.

Simplesse

No stranger to the profits that can be generated by fake foods, the NutraSweet Company unveiled its own fat substitute in 1988. Called Simplesse, this product is made of egg white or whey (a milk by-product) that has undergone a "microparticulation" process to turn it into tiny balls (50 billion per teaspoon) that mimic the texture of fat. Moreover, Simplesse is virtually cholesterol free and has just 1⅓ calories per gram, compared to 9 calories in a gram of real fat. Thus it can drastically reduce the calorie and fat content of products such as margarine, dips, spreads, and creamy dressings. Simplesse-laced ice cream, for example, has about half the usual calories.

Unlike Olestra, however, Simplesse breaks down when heated, so it can't be used in baked or fried foods. Thus, its uses are limited to frozen and uncooked products.

The FDA reviewed NutraSweet's data and has approved Simplesse for use in frozen desserts. However, CSPI has asked the FDA to require disclosure labels on any products containing Simplesse to warn people who are allergic to egg or milk proteins.

CSPI and other health agencies see additional potential drawbacks to fake fat. First, they question whether it really benefits those trying to lose weight. As with soft drinks containing NutraSweet (aspartame), many people may simply add them to their diet instead of using them as a substitute for high-calorie foods. And others may think this gives them a license to consume more, as is often the case with "diet" drinks.

Another concern is that people will indulge in formerly fatty junk foods, leaving little room for complex carbohydrates rich in essential vitamins, minerals, and fiber. The CSPI has asked the FDA to require nutritional impact studies to determine how fake fat alters the diet of those who use it.

Will Olestra and Simplesse be useful in reducing the fat and calorie content of the American diet, or will they, like artificial sweeteners, be another means for an overfed population to consume even more? We won't know until they've been on the market a while. And hopefully that won't happen on a widespread basis until they're proven safe.

Advances in Liposuction: Forecast for the 1990s

Liposuction, the renowned plastic surgery procedure, is likely to become even more popular in the 1990s. In the upcoming ten years, new technological refinements promise to make the operation simpler and more efficient, according to the American Society for Aesthetic Plastic Surgery, Inc.

"In the 1990s, people seeking an improved shape may be able to go to specially equipped body contouring centers where computer-controlled laser microchip devices will be used to suction off unwanted fat, achieving optimal results with minimal bruising, swelling, or discomfort," says Eugene Courtiss, M.D., assistant clinical professor of plastic surgery at Harvard Medical School.

The current method for removing excess fat deposits, such as those on the thighs, hips, or abdomen, is through manual manipulation by the surgeon of a long, hollow tube inserted beneath the skin and connected to a suction machine that literally vacuums away the fat. The primary danger is removal of too much fat.

In the next decade, computer technology will make liposuction easier and more precise, Dr. Courtiss predicted at a New York press briefing. "The patient will first have a magnetic resonant image (MRI) made of his or her body, through which the exact degree of fat will be measured and entered into a computer," says Dr. Courtiss. "A small incision will be made at the site where fat is to be removed and a laser microchip inserted. This microchip will move around inside the body, according to precise instructions given by the computer, suctioning out the unwanted fat. The patient will then be placed in a compression garment and sent home."

According to Dr. Courtiss, most of the technology is already in place, and the rest should be developed early in the 1990s. However, the criteria for determining who is a good candidate for liposuction is less likely to change in the near future, says Dr. Courtiss. People who get the best results from the procedure are healthy, no more than 10 pounds over their ideal weight, have resilient skin, and are under 40 years old. People who are between 40 and 60 can get acceptable results if they meet the other standards, but anyone over 60 who weighs more than 20 pounds over their ideal weight, smokes, has diabetes, phlebitis, cardiovascular disease, or poor skin tone is a poor candidate for liposuction. Talk to your doctor about your eligibility for this procedure.

Bigger Breasts: A Surprising Side Effect of Liposuction

Strange as it seems, some women who have lower-body liposuction actually experience breast enlargement afterward, say two dermatologic surgeons. Dr. Dwight Scarborough and Dr. Emil Bisaccia report that, among 30 female liposuction patients, 5 went up a full cup size, while another 11 reported increased breast fullness.

The doctors think this may be due to a combination of factors, including hormone levels and diet. But the most influential factor may be the location of the liposuction. "In women, the abdomen, thighs, and buttocks are 'fat banks'; that is, the places the body normally stores its fat reserves," says Dr. Scarborough. "We suspect that removing fat cells in those areas, which liposuction does, may induce the body to start storing fat somewhere else, such as the breasts."

Though none of their patients complained, not every woman would welcome this additional figure change, notes Dr. Scarborough. But right now, there is no sure way to predict which women's bodies will react this way. "One thing these women had in common was their age—most were in their mid-30s. But what may be more significant is that they each had a large amount of fat tissue removed—a full liter, which is about 4 cups."

Dr. Scarborough and Dr. Bisaccia are now measuring and evaluating caloric intake in another group of liposuction patients. They hope to learn why some women's breasts grow following the procedure and how to predict who will have this somewhat startling side effect.

After the Fat:
Taking the Skin out of Skinny

People who lose large amounts of weight often find that slenderness—like most things in life—has its pleasures and its disappointments.

One of the disappointments is loose skin. Some people find that they still don't have the taut, youthful body they see in fashion magazines. Instead, they have stretch marks and saggy skin. It doesn't happen to everyone. Younger skin has more elasticity and tends to "shrink" as you lose weight. Losing weight slowly gives your skin a greater chance to shrink back. And exercise tightens the underlying muscles, making the skin look better.

But you're especially susceptible to sagging skin if you're over 30 and have lost a lot of weight. Sometimes women who've gone through multiple pregnancies will also find that their skin and the underlying muscles have been stretched.

The extra skin isn't dangerous, but thousands of people a year are willing to pay the $2,000 to $6,000 (or more) it takes to "take in" their skin.

"Abdominoplasty" (also called "tummy tucks") is the most common form of skin surgery. Face, buttock, and breast lifts are also popular after weight loss. Some surgeons discourage tucks of hips, thighs, and upper arms because visible scarring can result. But, depending on the degree of sagging, a person may want to make the trade-off.

Verne C. Lanier, Jr., M.D., a North Carolina plastic surgeon, surveyed his patients, and found that 39 out of 50 (78 percent) felt such surgery after weight reduction improved their self-esteem.

Because the surgery is elective, not all insurance plans provide coverage. You may, however, be able to deduct the costs as a medical expense on your income tax return.

Is It in Your Thyroid or in Your Thighs?

You've probably seen news stories about First Lady Barbara Bush's treatment for a thyroid problem. One story mentioned weight gain as a symptom of an underactive thyroid, so *Prevention* decided to check it out.

For over 50 years, doctors mistakenly prescribed thyroid medication for obesity and other conditions. And despite dramatic changes in medical understanding of thyroid problems in recent years, "the myth that obesity is caused by thyroid insufficiency dies hard," writes Norman Schneeberg, M.D., a professor of endocrinology and metabolism at Hahnemann University Medical School in Philadelphia. "Most laypersons still believe it, and they often come to the physician seeking confirmation of a preconceived diagnosis."

Dr. Schneeberg has called pseudohypothyroidism (false underactive thyroid) the most common nondisease in the United States. In 1986 he reported that of the last 100 patients he examined for alleged thyroid failure, only 15 proved to be truly hypothyroid.

Just last year, the *Journal of the American Medical Association* published an editorial by David S. Cooper, M.D., of Johns Hopkins University School of Medicine, entitled "Thyroid Hormone Treatment: New Insights into an Old Therapy." The editorial noted that "previously well-accepted indications, e.g., obesity, infertility, fatigue, and [high cholesterol], are no longer valid." Dr. Cooper also reported that thyroid hormone preparations are "among the most commonly prescribed medications in this country."

And Ronald L. Smoyer, M.D., vice-president of the American Society of Bariatric Physicians, occasionally sees a new patient who reports having lost weight in the past on a "program" that turns out to have been small doses of thyroid extract. Years ago it was prescribed along with amphetamines and digoxin (which produces profound nausea). "I have to explain to them that we now know that such medications are not safe, effective ways to lose weight," says Dr. Smoyer. "Rainbow" diet programs (called that because they were multipill diets) containing thyroid were banned by the FDA a number of years ago.

Do You Need Thyroid Medication?

It's not hard to see why thyroid problems were thought to be a cause of obesity—the hormones secreted by the largest of our endocrine glands do play a critical role in regulating our metabolism. And moderate weight gain can be one of a group of symptoms that indicate an underactive thyroid. But that doesn't mean that thyroid medication should be routinely prescribed for weight loss.

Most overweight people do not have thyroid problems. And if you take too high a dose of thyroid hormone when your thyroid is functioning normally, you could become "hyperthyroid," and your heart rate, metabolism, and other organ systems will be speeded up. Sustained use of thyroid hormones could literally wear your body out early, making your bones thin and your heart weak and flabby.

Fortunately, tests developed in recent years to mea-sure thyroid function are much more sensitive and reliable than those used previously. These tests have enabled phy-sicians to understand more clearly how thyroid hormones work and how to diagnose and treat thyroid diseases accurately.

And while thyroid problems are not usually the cause of obesity, they are more common for women. The Amer-ican Thyroid Association reports that about seven million Americans have been diagnosed with thyroid disorders. And they estimate that an additional three million people, mostly women and the elderly, suffer from unrecognized thyroid problems. Four to five times as many women are affected as men, and the problem is more common and more difficult to diagnose in the elderly. Experts estimate that one in every eight women over age 50 has evidence of the earliest stages of hypothyroidism.

The Symptoms

Basically, there are two types of thyroid problems—overactive, or *hyper*thyroidism, and underactive, or *hypo*-thyroidism. Barbara Bush suffers from Graves' disease, a condition that causes hyperthyroidism. Symptoms include speedy metabolism leading to increased appetite and weight loss, weakness, damp skin and palms, irritability, feeling warm even when it's cool, tremors, and bulging eyes. Mrs. Bush lost weight during her illness and then, after treatment, regained it.

But it's hypothyroidism that may include moderate weight gain as a symptom, along with loss of appetite, lethargy, feeling cold, memory impairment, dry skin and palms, constipation, and menstrual irregularities. These symptoms can sometimes be recognized as due to thyroid failure but are more often mistaken for normal aging or attributed to diseases of other organ systems.

If you have gradually gained some weight without any apparent changes in your diet or activity level, and you have any of the other symptoms described above, you might want to ask your doctor to test your thyroid. The most sensitive initial test measures your TSH—thyroid-stimulating hormone—level.

The Causes

Hypothyroidism is two to three times more common than hyperthyroidism, but the main cause of both is believed to be autoimmune disease—where the body's immune system mistakenly attacks its own cells as if they were foreign invaders. Iodine deficiency can also cause hypothyroidism, but this has become nonexistent in the

United States since the addition of iodine to table salt.

Like other autoimmune diseases, thyroid problems may be inherited, and they may appear after a major period of stress (perhaps including surviving the rigors of a presidential campaign).

Interestingly, severe dieting or eating disorders like anorexia may mimic some of the symptoms of hypothyroidism. Blood levels of the thyroid hormone decrease, and metabolism slows down. However, unlike true hypothyroidism, this is a temporary condition that will disappear when you stop fasting.

Other causes of thyroid dysfunction are use of certain drugs, including lithium for manic depression; iodine in the form of kelp, used as a health-food supplement; and a drug called amiodirone, used to treat cardiac arrhythmias. Problems with the pituitary gland, which controls the thyroid, may disrupt its functioning but are uncommon. Also, surgery or radioactive iodine used to treat hyperthyroidism can result in the opposite problem—hypothyroidism.

The Treatment

Fortunately, most thyroid problems respond very well to proper diagnosis and treatment. Symptoms of hypothyroidism in particular usually disappear completely when the patient takes daily doses of a synthetic thyroid hormone called levothyroxine. Although most patients will have to continue this medication for their entire life, there are usually no side effects when it is given in the correct dose.

Remember Cal-Ban?
By the Editors of *Lose Weight Naturally* Newsletter

Imagine our surprise (and dismay) when we opened our local morning paper and found an ad for the old weight-loss fraud Cal-Ban 3000. Since *Lose Weight Naturally* newsletter did a line-by-line analysis of a Cal-Ban ad, Anderson Pharmaceuticals, the company that peddles the stuff, has taken some of the more law-breaking phrases—as well as their own name—out of its promos. They've also added a few waffle words like "appears" and "according to one informed source." But they're still selling the same old guar gum, outrageously overpriced and still unproven as a weight-loss aid.

Our red-faced local newspaper reported the day after the ad ran that the U.S. Postal Service still bans mail delivery to Anderson. The paper broke its policy of not taking ads like this in part because of the "money-back" guarantee. Only later did they learn that, since you can't write to the company, you can't take advantage of their offer to return the empty bottle for a full refund. (The ad doesn't even list an address where you can send the bottle.)

The other reason the paper took the ad was because it listed two local pharmacies that stock Cal-Ban. One pulled it off their shelves after a local doctor called and pointed out that Cal-Ban's claims were illegal. But the other, apparently of the "Profit before Honor" school of business, was selling the stuff hand over fist the morning the ad appeared.

We doubt that this was an isolated incident that just happened to pop up right in our newsletter's backyard. Even being forbidden to use the mail doesn't appear to have deterred Cal-Ban's distributor. You may find it being advertised and sold in your area, too. Don't think this means they've cleaned up their act and now are selling a product that works. They haven't, and it doesn't.

However, a case of a guar gum tablet controlling food intake too well was reported in the *New England Journal of Medicine.* Two Veterans Administration Medical Center doctors in Minneapolis treated an overweight man who had been unable to swallow anything for 12 hours after taking a guar gum and grapefruit fiber diet aid. When they

228 The Diet Detective

looked down his throat with an endoscope, they found
that the tablet had swelled and blocked his esophagus.
The endoscope itself broke up the impacted tablet. The
doctors wryly observed that such diet pills are seldom as
effective as this one.

Arm Yourself against Diet Fraud

Now you know about Cal-Ban 3000. This perennial
weight-loss fraud is often down, but apparently never out—
despite the fact that the U.S. Postal Service has forbidden
Cal-Ban's parent company to use the mail service.

Cal-Ban's dogged persistence raises an important issue about the $33-billion weight-loss industry in this coun-
try: There are a heck of a lot of people out there ready and
willing to take your money while offering something unproven and costly—or even dangerous—in return.

Even some of the more established programs are apparently not without risk. New evidence indicates that even
hospital-supervised fasting programs may be worse than
ineffective.

It's hard to keep on top of the diet dangers out there,
especially because some of the claims are *so* tempting.
Instant, painless, weight loss. The ultimate fantasy.

The only way to resist these beguiling temptations is
to build some healthy skepticism into your brain's operating structure. You can cultivate that skepticism by asking
questions, and not accepting simple answers.

Jane White, Ph.D., professor at Catholic University of
America's School of Nursing, has studied the psychology
of weight loss. She recommends asking the following three
questions as the first step toward arming yourself against
diet fraud.

1. Who is running the program? Are they trained
professionals? How much experience do they have?

2. What kind of follow-up does the program offer for after weight loss? Most people can lose weight, but few can keep it off. "So don't bother asking about success rates," says Dr. White. "Instead, find out about the follow-up period. How long is it? What does it consist of? Structure and support are important, especially to those who have a background of obesity."

3. Does the program include nutrition, exercise, and behavior modification? All three aspects of dieting are necessary, says Dr. White. "Some types of liquid diets and surgery may result in dramatic weight loss, but if the dieter receives no education or support to change eating habits, he or she may regain the weight."

It's undisputable: People who've successfully maintained their weight loss, often after years of yo-yo-ing, have done it by changing their lifestyle. Weight loss is a step-by-step process of physical, emotional and spiritual change and healing.

In fact, the most successful weight loss is always accompanied by personal growth—and we all know how long that takes. So be careful and critical of any weight-loss program or product that doesn't address these crucial components.

CHAPTER

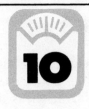

THE FAT-FIGHTER'S COMPANION

America's Changing Its Tastes

According to a survey of over 1,100 consumers, Americans today are more concerned than ever about dietary fat. We all know (or at least we should) that less than 30 percent of our calories should come from fat. And we know that to keep our intake below 30 percent, each of the foods we choose should be low in fat.

Our concerns about food are reflected in today's marketplace, where there's an increasing demand for products that are low in cholesterol and fat—without compromising taste and nutrition.

And the food industry is responding. Supermarkets today have a wider and wider variety of foods that are not just reduced fat but are completely fat free! Even more low-fat products are currently in test markets around the country and will be appearing on your supermarket shelves soon.

One example of a new low-fat or no-fat food is Yog-lacé, an "I Can't Believe It's Yogurt" product. It contains *no* fat and *no* cholesterol and is only a tasty 10 calories per ounce. Several other nonfat frozen yogurts are a welcome taste treat for the weight conscious, although they are slightly higher in calories than Yoglacé.

Buyer Beware: Not All "Light" or "Lean" Foods Are Low-Fat

With all the new "lighter" foods popping up, it can be very confusing to navigate around the claims on the packaging. Some manufacturers are more than willing to take advantage of you. For example, nutritional analysis revealed that one cake product with the word "light" written across the package was loaded with fat and calories. When questioned, the company claimed that by "light" it meant the cake had a light and creamy taste!

There's also a popular "light and smooth" frozen dessert out there that is almost as fattening as regular ice cream!

So now more than ever, it's important to get the facts about fat. That's why we've compiled this updated and expanded reference guide. It lists the calories, grams of fat, percentage of calories from fat, and (where appropriate) the predominant type of fat for hundreds of common foods.

When looking at a particular food, the single most important number is the percentage of calories from fat. Because it's given as a percentage, the figure won't change for different serving sizes and you can easily compare one food on the chart to another. This will help you select the one that's best.

It's also important to know that some types of fat are better for you than others. As a rule, you should try to replace saturated fats with polyunsaturated and monounsaturated fats. Whenever possible, we've indicated which type of fat prevails in the foods. S stands for saturated (and stay away), P for polyunsaturated, and M for monounsaturated.

THE FAT FIGHTER'S INDEX

FOOD	PORTION	TOTAL CALORIES	FAT (g)	CALORIES FROM FAT (%)
BAKED GOODS				♦
Biscuit	1 (2″)	99	4.2	38
Bread				
Cracked wheat	1 slice (1 oz.)	66	0.9	12
"Lite" or diet	1 slice (1 oz.)	40	1.0	18
Oat bran	1 slice (1 oz.)	65	1.0	14
Pita pocket	1 (1.3 oz.)	105	0.6	5
Wheat	1 slice (1 oz.)	66	1.3	18
White and mixed grain	1 slice (1 oz.)	64	0.9	13
Croutons	0.5 oz.	70	3.0	39
Muffins				
Blueberry	1 (2⅝″)	110	4.0	33
Bran	1 (2⅝″)	112	5.1	41
Corn	1 (2⅝″)	121	4.0	30
English	1	118	0.8	6
English, oat bran	1	185	1.0	4
Rolls				
Brown 'n' serve	1 (1 oz.)	85	2.0	21
Hard	1 (1.75 oz.)	155	2.0	12
Hoagie	1 (4.75 oz.)	390	4.0	9

FOOD	PORTION	TOTAL CALORIES	FAT (g)	CALORIES FROM FAT (%)
BREAKFAST FOODS				♦
Bacon, fried or broiled	1 slice	36	3.1	77 S,M
Bagel (see Delicatessen Foods on page 242)				
Breakfast meat strips	3 strips	80	6.0	68
Canadian bacon, grilled	1 slice	43	2.0	41 M
Cereals				
Corn bran	1 cup	124	1.3	9
Cornflakes	1 cup	98	0.1	1
Cream of Wheat	1 cup	144	0.6	3

NOTE: S = saturated; P = polyunsaturated; M = monounsaturated

FOOD	PORTION	TOTAL CALORIES	FAT (g)	CALORIES FROM FAT (%)
Granola, homemade	½ cup	298	16.6	50 M,P
Granola, purchased	½ cup	252	9.8	35 S
Grits	1 cup	146	0.5	3
"O-shaped" oats	1 cup	91	1.1	11
Oat flakes	1 cup	177	0.7	4
Oatmeal	1 cup	145	2.4	15
Rice, crispy	1 cup	109	11.9	11
Rice, puffed	1 cup	56	0.1	2
Shredded wheat	1 cup	83–169	0.6	5
Shredded wheat w/raisins	1 cup	150	0.7	4
Wheat bran flakes	1 cup	146	0.7	5
Wheat bran flakes w/raisins	1 cup	169	0.8	4
Croissant, frozen	1	109	6.1	50
Danish pastry, plain	1	250	13.6	49 S
Doughnut, yeast, glazed	1	205	11.2	49 M
Egg				
Raw or poached	1	79	5.6	63 S
Scrambled w/milk and butter	1	95	7.1	67 S
Substitute*	¼ cup	25	0.0	0
White	1	16	0.0	0
Eggs, sausage, and hash browns, frozen	5.5 oz. pkg.	360	28.0	70
French toast				
Frozen	1 slice	85–135	2.5–7.0	27–48
Homemade	1 slice	153	6.7	40
Instant breakfast drink	1 cup	280	8.0	26
Pancake				
Frozen	1	80	3.5	39
Mix	1	58	2.1	32
Pastry, toaster	1	196	5.8	26
Sausage links, low-fat	2–3	160	11.5	66

* Read labels carefully. Some foods in this category may be surprisingly high in fat.

(continued)

THE FAT FIGHTER'S INDEX—Continued

FOOD	PORTION	TOTAL CALORIES	FAT (g)	CALORIES FROM FAT (%)
BREAKFAST FOODS—Continued				♦
Scrambled eggs and home fries, frozen	4.74 oz. pkg.	280	21.0	68
Waffle				
Frozen	1	106	4.8	31
Homemade	1	245	12.6	46
Mix	1	205	8.0	35
Wheat germ, toasted	1 Tbsp.	27	0.3	25 P
COMBINATION FOODS: DINNERS				♦
Beef cannelloni, light, frozen	9.6 oz.	260	10.0	35
Beef dinner, frozen	12 oz.	320	9.0	25
Beef teriyaki, light, frozen	8 oz.	240	3.0	11
Cheese cannelloni, light, frozen	9.1 oz.	270	10.0	33
Chicken w/broccoli, light, frozen	9.5 oz.	290	11.0	34
Chicken cacciatore, frozen	11.2 oz.	310	11.0	32
Chicken chow mein, light, frozen	11.2 oz.	250	5.0	18
Chicken dinner, frozen	11.5 oz.	660	33.0	45
Chicken divan, frozen	8.5 oz.	335	22.0	59
Chicken parmigiana, frozen	11.5 oz.	400	20.0	45
Chicken w/vegetables and rice, light	8.5 oz.	270	8.0	27
Fish and chips, frozen	7.9 oz.	500	30.0	54
Kraft Macaroni & Cheese (dry mix)				
Made w/milk and margarine	¼ pkg.	290	13.0	40
Made w/skim milk and butter sprinkles	¼ pkg.	207	2.0	9
Lasagna, frozen	10.5 oz.	385	14.0	33
Lasagna Florentine, light	11.2 oz.	280	5.0	16

FOOD	PORTION	TOTAL CALORIES	FAT (g)	CALORIES FROM FAT (%)
Lipton Pasta & Sauce (dry mix)				
Cheddar Broccoli				
Made w/milk and butter	¼ pkg.	200	9.0	41
Made w/skim milk				
and butter sprinkles	¼ pkg.	155	2.0	12
Creamy Garlic				
Made w/milk and butter	¼ pkg.	210	10.0	43
Made w/skim milk				
and butter sprinkles	¼ pkg.	155	3.0	17
Lobster Newburg	6.5 oz.	350	29.0	75
Manicotti w/cheese, frozen	8.5 oz.	310	13.0	38
Meatballs w/noodles, frozen	11 oz.	475	27.0	51
Meat loaf dinner, frozen	11 oz.	412	23.7	52
Mueller's Chef Series (dry mix)				
Garlic & Butter				
Made w/butter	½ cup	170	7.0	37
Made w/1½ tsp.				
butter sprinkles	½ cup	123	2.0	15
Alfredo				
Made w/butter	½ cup	190	9.0	43
Made w/1½ tsp.				
butter sprinkles	½ cup	123	3.0	22
Salad Bar Pasta				
Made w/2 Tbsp. oil	½ cup	140	5.0	22
Ronzoni Classic Pasta				
Dishes (dry mix)				
Fettucine Alfredo				
Made w/milk and butter	½ cup	200	10.0	45
Made w/skim milk				
and butter sprinkles	½ cup	144	3.0	19
Four Cheese				
Made w/milk and butter	½ cup	200	9.0	41
Made w/skim milk				
and butter sprinkles	½ cup	144	2.0	13

(continued)

THE FAT FIGHTER'S INDEX—Continued

FOOD	PORTION	TOTAL CALORIES	FAT (g)	CALORIES FROM FAT (%)

COMBINATION FOODS: DINNERS—Continued ♦

FOOD	PORTION	TOTAL CALORIES	FAT (g)	CALORIES FROM FAT (%)
Salisbury steak, frozen	11 oz.	390	24.6	57
Scallops Mariner, frozen	10.2 oz.	400	16.0	36
Shells w/beef, frozen	9 oz.	290	11.0	34
Shells w/cheese, frozen	9 oz.	320	14.0	39
Shells w/chicken, frozen	9 oz.	400	22.0	50
Shrimp creole, light, frozen	10 oz.	200	2.0	9
Sirloin tips, frozen	11.5 oz.	390	18.0	42
Sweet and sour chicken, frozen	11.2 oz.	460	22.0	43
Tuna w/noodles, frozen	5.7 oz.	200	9.0	41
Turkey breast, premium dinner, frozen	11.2 oz.	470	24.0	45
Turkey dinner, w/potatoes, frozen	11.5 oz.	340	10.0	27
Vegetable lasagna	11 oz.	400	24.0	54
Yankee pot roast, frozen	11 oz.	360	15.0	38
Zucchini lasagna, light	11 oz.	260	7.0	24

COMBINATION FOODS: ENTRÉES ♦

FOOD	PORTION	TOTAL CALORIES	FAT (g)	CALORIES FROM FAT (%)
Barbecue chicken, light, frozen	8 oz.	300	6.0	18
Beef burgundy, frozen	5 oz.	144	5.0	31
Beef chop suey, homemade	1 cup	300	17.0	51 S
Beef potpie	4 oz.	279	16.2	52 M
Beef stew w/vegetables	1 cup	220	11.0	45 S,M
Beef Stroganoff, frozen	5.9 oz.	192	8.0	38
Chicken, glazed, light, frozen	8 oz.	230	4.0	16
Chicken à la king	1 cup	470	34.0	65 M,S
Chicken chow mein, homemade	1 cup	255	10.0	35 S
Chicken w/dumplings, frozen	1 oz	31	1.3	38 M
Chicken Kiev, frozen	8.2 oz.	500	30.0	54
Chicken potpie, homemade	4 oz.	273	15.2	51 M,S
Chili con carne, canned	1 cup	340	16.0	42 M,S

FOOD	PORTION	TOTAL CALORIES	FAT (g)	CALORIES FROM FAT (%)
Creamed chipped beef, frozen	5.5 oz.	235	16.0	61
Enchilada	8 oz.	396	20.9	48
Fettuccine Alfredo, frozen	5 oz.	270	18.0	60
Fish almandine, frozen	4 oz.	236	17.0	65
Fish Florentine, light, frozen	9 oz.	240	9.0	34
Hamburger w/bacon and cheese	5.3 oz.	464	27.3	53
Macaroni and cheese, light, frozen	9 oz.	300	9.0	27
Meat loaf w/celery and onions	3 oz.	213	13.9	59 M,S
Noodles Romanoff, frozen	4 oz.	170	9.0	48
Ravioli w/beef, canned	3 oz.	83	1.7	19
Seafood gumbo, frozen	4 oz.	40	0.4	9
Sole w/lemon sauce, light, frozen	4 oz.	262	21.0	72
Sole, light, frozen	5 oz.	293	18.0	55
Spaghetti, canned	1 cup	190	2.0	9 S
Spaghetti w/sauce and cheese, homemade	1 cup	260	9.0	31 S
Spareribs w/BBQ sauce, frozen	4 oz.	216	13.2	55 S,M
Turkey, sliced, light, frozen	8 oz.	230	5.0	20
Turkey w/gravy, frozen	1 cup	160	6.3	35 M,S
Turkey pie, frozen	10 oz.	460	26.0	51
Veal parmigiana, frozen	7.5 oz.	296	14.0	43
Veal steak, light, frozen	11 oz.	280	8.0	26

CONDIMENTS ◆

FOOD	PORTION	TOTAL CALORIES	FAT (g)	CALORIES FROM FAT (%)
Horseradish, prepared	1 Tbsp.	6	0	0
Ketchup	1 Tbsp.	15	0.1	6
Mayonnaise	1 Tbsp.	99	11.0	100 P
Mayonnaise, low-calorie	1 Tbsp.	40	4.0	90
Mayonnaise-style spread dressing	1 Tbsp.	60	5.2	79 P

(continued)

FOOD	PORTION	TOTAL CALORIES	FAT (g)	CALORIES FROM FAT (%)
CONDIMENTS—Continued				◆
Mustard				
Brown	1 Tbsp.	14	1.0	62
Yellow	1 Tbsp.	15	0.3	18
Olives, green or black	5	22	2.9	100 M
Pickles				
Dill	1	5	0.1	18
Sweet	1 small	20	0.1	5
Relish	1 oz.	33	0.01	3
Soy sauce	1 Tbsp.	11	0	0
Tamari sauce	1 Tbsp.	11	0.1	2 P
Teriyaki sauce	1 Tbsp.	15	0	0
DAIRY PRODUCTS				◆
Buttermilk	1 cup	99	2.2	20 S
Cheeses				
American, processed	1 oz.	106	8.9	75 S
American, singles	1 oz.	45	2.0	40
Blue	1 oz.	60	4.9	73 S
Brick	1 oz.	105	8.4	70
Brie	1 oz.	95	7.9	74 S
Camembert	1 oz.	85	6.9	71
Cheddar	1 oz.	114	9.4	74 S
Cheshire	1 oz.	110	8.7	69
Colby	1 oz.	112	9.1	73 S
Cottage	¼ cup	58	2.5	39 S
Cottage, low-fat (1%)	¼ cup	41	0.5	13
Cream	1 oz.	99	9.9	90 S
Edam	1 oz.	101	7.9	69
Feta	1 oz.	75	6.0	72 S
Fontina	1 oz.	110	8.8	71
Gouda	1 oz.	101	7.8	68

FOOD	PORTION	TOTAL CALORIES	FAT (g)	CALORIES FROM FAT (%)
Gruyère	1 oz.	117	9.2	69
Monterey Jack	1 oz.	106	8.6	73
Monterey Jack, light	1 oz.	80	6.0	68
Mozzarella, part-skim	1 oz.	72	4.5	56
Mozzarella, whole-milk	1 oz.	80	6.1	69
Muenster	1 oz.	104	8.5	72
Neufchâtel	1 oz.	74	6.6	79
Parmesan, grated	1 Tbsp.	29	1.9	59
Provolone	1 oz.	100	7.6	66
Ricotta, part-skim	¼ cup	85	4.9	52
Ricotta, whole-milk	¼ cup	107	8.0	67
Romano	1 oz.	110	7.6	61
Roquefort	1 oz.	105	8.7	73
Swiss	1 oz.	107	7.8	65 S
Swiss, light	1 oz.	50	2.0	36
Cream				
Half-and-half	1 Tbsp.	20	1.7	79
Light	1 Tbsp.	29	2.9	89
Heavy, whipping	1 Tbsp.	51	5.5	97 S
Milk				
Chocolate	1 cup	208	8.5	37 S
Evaporated	1 Tbsp.	21	1.2	51 S
Evaporated skim	1 Tbsp.	12	0.1	2
Low-fat (1%)	1 cup	102	2.6	23 S
Skim	1 cup	86	0.4	5 S
Whole	1 cup	150	8.2	49 S
Nondairy creamers				
Regular	1 Tbsp.	10	1.0	80 S
Diet	1 packet	10	0	0
Nondairy whipped				
topping, frozen	1 Tbsp.	15	1.2	72 S
Sour cream				
Cultured	1 Tbsp.	31	3.0	88 S
Imitation	1 Tbsp.	28	2.6	84

(continued)

241

THE FAT FIGHTER'S INDEX—Continued

FOOD	PORTION	TOTAL CALORIES	FAT (g)	CALORIES FROM FAT (%)
DAIRY PRODUCTS—Continued				◆
Yogurt				
Low-fat	1 cup	144	3.5	22
Nonfat	1 cup	127	0.4	3
Whole-milk	1 cup	139	7.4	48 S
Yogurt cheese	1 oz.	30	0.6	18
Yogurt drink	1 cup	190	4.0	19
DELICATESSEN FOODS				◆
Bagels				
Egg or plain	1 (2 oz.)	163	1.4	8
W/cream cheese	1 (2 oz.)	361	21.1	53
W/lox and onion	1 (2 oz.)	243	3.9	15
Luncheon meats				
Bologna, pork	1 oz.	70	5.6	72 M,S
Corned beef	1 oz.	71	5.4	68 M,S
Ham, baked	1 oz.	52	3.0	52 M,S
Ham, turkey	1 oz.	37	1.4	36
Ham and cheese loaf	1 oz.	73	5.7	71 M,S
Liverwurst	1 oz.	93	8.1	78 M,S
Olive loaf	1 oz.	67	4.7	63 M,S
Pastrami, beef	1 oz.	99	8.3	75 M,S
Pastrami, turkey	1 oz.	40	2.1	46 S
Pickle/pimiento loaf	1 oz.	74	6.0	73 M,S
Salami, cooked beef	1 oz.	72	5.7	72
Salami, hard	1 oz.	116	9.6	74 M,S
Salads				
Chef's	average	722	56.1	70
Chef's, no dressing	average	344	20.1	53
Chicken	⅔ cup	509	39.0	69
Coleslaw	½ cup	127	11.1	79
Cucumber	¾ cup	43	2.2	47

FOOD	PORTION	TOTAL CALORIES	FAT (g)	CALORIES FROM FAT (%)
Egg	½ cup	425	41.0	86
Greek, w/feta cheese	average	377	21.5	51
Macaroni	½ cup	286	25.1	79
Pickled cabbage	½ cup	70	6.1	79
Potato, German	¾ cup	164	3.3	18
Potato, w/mayonnaise	¾ cup	288	18.9	59
Tuna	⅓ cup	306	26.1	77
Sandwiches				
Grilled cheese	1	440	31.0	63
Ham and cheese on rye w/mustard and mayonnaise	1	615	37.7	55
Hero	1	1,154	62.2	49
Pastrami, beef, on rye	1	541	36.0	60
Pastrami, turkey, on whole wheat	1	297	11.6	35
Reuben, grilled, on rye	1	835	59.5	64
Roast beef w/horseradish on rye	1	444	18.8	38
Roast beef w/mayonnaise, tomato, lettuce on rye	1	576	35.1	55
Tuna/cheese melt	1	640	48.2	68
Turkey club on white	1	626	33.5	48
Turkey club on whole wheat	1	357	14.3	36

DESSERTS AND SWEETS ◆

Brownies				
Fudge, microwave	1 oz.	180	9.0	45
W/nuts, no icing, homemade	1 oz.	135	8.5	57 S
W/nuts, no icing, mix	1 oz.	121	5.7	42 S
Iced	1 oz.	105	5.0	43 M,S
Candy				
Caramel, plain and chocolate	1 oz.	115	3.0	23 S

(continued)

THE FAT FIGHTER'S INDEX—Continued

FOOD	PORTION	TOTAL CALORIES	FAT (g)	CALORIES FROM FAT (%)
DESSERTS AND SWEETS—Continued				◆
Candy—*continued*				
Chocolate bar w/peanuts	1 oz.	154	10.8	63
Chocolate-covered peanuts	1 oz.	160	12.0	68 S
Fudge	1 oz.	115	3.0	23 S
Gumdrops	1 oz.	100	0	0
Jelly beans	1	7	0	0
Milk chocolate bar	1 oz.	145	9.0	56 S
Semisweet chocolate bar	1 oz.	144	10.2	64 S
Cakes				
Angel food, mix	2 oz.	142	0.1	1
Coffee cake, mix	2.5 oz.	230	7.0	27 S
Cheesecake	3 oz.	257	16.3	57
Cheesecake, low-calorie	4 oz.	180	6.0	30
Devil's-food, iced, mix	2.5 oz.	235	8.0	31 S
Pineapple upside-down, homemade	2.5 oz.	221	8.5	35
Pound, homemade	2 oz.	275	17.2	56 S
Sponge, homemade	2.3 oz.	188	3.1	15 S
Cookies				
Chocolate chip, homemade	1 small	46	2.7	52 M,P
Chocolate chip, mix	1 small	50	2.4	44 M,S
Chocolate/vanilla sandwich	1 small	50	2.3	41 S
Fig bar	1 average	53	1.0	16 S
Fudge	1 small	25	1.0	36
Gingersnap, homemade	1 small	34	1.6	42 S
Macaroon	1 average	90	4.5	45
Peanut butter, homemade	1 average	59	3.3	50
Peanut butter, mix	1 small	50	2.6	48
Vanilla wafer	1 small	19	0.6	29 M
Custard, baked	1 cup	305	15.0	46 S
Dessert sauces				
Butterscotch, homemade	1 Tbsp.	94	4.3	42 S

FOOD	PORTION	TOTAL CALORIES	FAT (g)	CALORIES FROM FAT (%)
Chocolate, homemade	1 Tbsp.	55	2.3	38 S
Hot fudge, homemade	1 Tbsp.	80	2.6	29 S
Eclair, custard-filled, iced	3.5 oz.	239	13.6	51
Gelatin, fruit-flavored	1 cup	161	3.1	17
Gingerbread, mix	2.2 oz.	175	4.0	21 S
Ice cream				
Caramel sundae	6 oz.	328	9.9	27
Hot fudge sundae	6 oz.	312	10.9	31
Soft	1 cup	377	22.5	54 S
10% fat	1 cup	269	14.3	48 S
Vanilla	1 cup	349	23.7	61 S
Ice milk				
Soft	1 cup	223	4.6	19 S
Vanilla	1 cup	184	5.6	28 S
Marshmallows	1 oz.	90	0	0
Mousse, chocolate, homemade	⅔ cup	445	35.7	72 S
Pies				
Apple, homemade	5 oz.	323	13.6	38 S
Banana cream, homemade	4.5 oz.	285	12.0	38 S
Blueberry, homemade	5 oz.	325	15.0	42 S
Cherry, homemade	5 oz.	350	15.0	39 S
Chocolate cream, homemade	3.5 oz.	264	15.1	52
Custard, homemade	4.5 oz.	285	14.0	44 S
Lemon meringue, homemade	4 oz.	300	11.2	34 S
Pumpkin, homemade	4.5 oz.	275	15.0	49 S
Puddings				
Chocolate, homemade	1 cup	385	12.0	28 S
Rice, w/raisins, homemade	1 cup	387	8.2	19
Tapioca, homemade	1 cup	220	8.0	33 S
Vanilla, homemade	1 cup	285	10.0	32 S
Sherbet, orange	1 cup	270	3.8	13 S
Syrup, chocolate flavor	1 oz.	83	0.3	4
Tofutti	1 cup	210	12.0	51

(continued)

FOOD	PORTION	TOTAL CALORIES	FAT (g)	CALORIES FROM FAT (%)

DESSERTS AND SWEETS—*Continued* ◆

FOOD	PORTION	TOTAL CALORIES	FAT (g)	CALORIES FROM FAT (%)
Turnovers				
Apple	1 oz.	85	4.7	50
Lemon	1 oz.	93	5.0	49
Yogurt, frozen, fruit flavor	1 cup	216	2.0	8

FAST FOODS ◆

FOOD	PORTION	TOTAL CALORIES	FAT (g)	CALORIES FROM FAT (%)
Breakfast foods				
Burger King bagel				
w/egg and cheese	1	387	14.0	33
Burger King bagel w/sausage	1	621	36.0	52
Burger King Croissan'wich	1	304	19.0	56
Burger King Croissan'wich				
w/bacon	1	355	24.0	61
Burger King				
french toast sticks	1 order	499	29.0	52
Burger King Great Danish	1	500	36.0	6
Burger King scrambled egg				
and sausage platter	1	702	52.0	67
McDonald's biscuit				
w/biscuit spread	1	260	12.7	44 M,S
McDonald's biscuit w/egg	1	529	35.3	60 M,S
McDonald's biscuit w/sausage	1	440	29.1	60 M,S
McDonald's Egg McMuffin	1	293	11.9	37 M,S
McDonald's English muffin				
w/butter	1	169	4.6	24 S
McDonald's hotcakes w/syrup	1 order	413	9.2	20 S,M
Roy Rogers breakfast crescent	1	401	12.0	27
Roy Rogers breakfast crescent				
w/bacon	1	431	13.9	29
Roy Rogers pancake platter	1	452	7.5	15

FOOD	PORTION	TOTAL CALORIES	FAT (g)	CALORIES FROM FAT (%)
Wendy's breakfast sandwich	1	370	19.0	46
Wendy's french toast	2 slices	400	19.0	43
Wendy's omelet w/cheese and ham	1	290	21.0	65
Wendy's sausage patty w/gravy	1 patty	640	54.0	76
Wendy's sausage patty w/out gravy	1 patty	200	18.0	81
Chicken and fish				
Arthur Treacher's chicken	4.8 oz.	369	21.6	53 P
Arthur Treacher's fish	5.2 oz.	355	19.8	50 P
Burger King Chicken Tenders	6 pieces	204	10.0	44
McDonald's Chicken McNuggets	4 oz.	288	16.3	51 P
Roy Rogers chicken breast	average	324	18.0	50
Roy Rogers chicken leg	average	117	6.0	46
Wendy's chicken nuggets	6 pieces	310	21.0	61
Desserts				
Burger King apple pie	1	305	12.0	35
McDonald's apple pie	1	262	14.8	51 M,S
McDonald's cone, soft serve	3 oz.	144	4.5	28 M,S
McDonald's sundae, hot fudge	6 oz.	313	9.4	27 S,M
Mexican foods				
Taco Bell burrito, bean	1	357	10.2	26 S
Taco Bell burrito, beef	1	403	17.3	39 S
Taco Bell chili	9 oz.	230	9.0	35
Taco Bell taco	1	183	10.8	53 S
Taco Bell taco bellgrande	1	355	23.0	59 S
Taco Bell taco, light	1	410	28.8	63 S
Taco Bell tostada	1	243	11.1	41 S

(continued)

THE FAT FIGHTER'S INDEX—Continued

FOOD	PORTION	TOTAL CALORIES	FAT (g)	CALORIES FROM FAT (%)
FAST FOODS—*Continued*				◆
Salads				
Arby's cashew chicken salad	13.4 oz.	590	37.0	56 P,M
Arby's chef's salad	11.1 oz.	210	11.0	47 S,M
Arby's garden salad	8.8 oz.	149	8.6	54 S
Arby's side salad	5.4 oz.	25	0	0
Burger King chef's salad	9.8 oz.	178	9.0	46 S,M
Burger King chunky chicken salad	9.2 oz.	142	4.0	25
Burger King garden salad	8 oz.	95	5.0	47 S
Burger King side salad	4.8 oz.	25	0	0
Hardee's chef's salad	10.5 oz.	240	15.0	56 S,M
Hardee's garden salad	8.6 oz.	210	14.0	60 S,M
Long John Silver's ocean chef's salad	8.4 oz.	150	5.0	30 S,M
Long John Silver's seafood salad	9.9 oz.	230	5.0	20 P,M
McDonald's chef's salad	10.1 oz.	230	13.6	51 M,S
McDonald's chunky chicken salad	8.9 oz.	140	3.4	19 M
McDonald's garden salad	7.6 oz.	110	6.6	57 M,S
McDonald's side salad	4.1 oz.	60	3.3	45 M,S
Taco Bell taco salad	20.5 oz.	905	61.0	60 S
Wendy's chef's salad	11.8 oz.	180	9.0	45
Wendy's garden salad	9.9 oz.	102	5.0	44
Wendy's taco salad	28.3 oz.	660	37.0	51
Sandwiches				
Arby's Bacon 'n Cheddar Deluxe roast beef	1	526	35.7	61
Arby's fish fillet	1	580	30.9	48
Arby's roast-beef	1	350	15.0	39
Arby's Super	1	501	21.7	39
Arthur Treacher's chicken	1	413	19.2	42 P

FOOD	PORTION	TOTAL CALORIES	FAT (g)	CALORIES FROM FAT (%)
Arthur Treacher's fish	1	440	24.0	49 P
Burger King bacon				
double cheeseburger	1	510	31.0	55
Burger King chicken specialty	1	688	40.0	52
Burger King Whaler	1	488	27.0	50
Burger King Whopper	1	630	36.0	51
Burger King Whopper w/cheese	1	711	43.0	54
McDonald's Big Mac	1	562	32.4	52 M,S
McDonald's Fillet o' Fish	1	442	26.1	53 P,M
McDonald's hamburger	1	257	9.5	33 M,S
McDonald's McD.L.T.	1	674	42.1	56 M,S
McDonald's McLean Deluxe	1	320	10.0	28 M,S
McDonald's McLean Deluxe				
w/cheese	1	370	14.0	34 M,S
McDonald's Quarter Pounder	1	414	20.7	45 M,S
McDonald's Quarter Pounder				
w/cheese	1	517	29.2	51 M,S
Roy Rogers roast beef	1	317	9.9	28
Roy Rogers roast beef w/cheese	1	467	19.7	38
Wendy's Bacon Swiss burger	1	710	44.0	56
Wendy's Big Classic Double	1	680	39.0	52
Wendy's chicken	1	430	19.0	40
Shakes				
Burger King vanilla	regular	321	10.0	28
McDonald's vanilla	regular	354	10.2	26 S,M
Side orders				
Burger King french fries	regular	227	13.0	52
Burger King onion rings	regular	274	16.0	53
McDonald's french fries	regular	220	11.5	47 S,M
Wendy's baked potato	8.8 oz.	250	2.0	7
Wendy's baked potato				
w/broccoli and cheese	12.9 oz.	500	25.0	45
Wendy's baked potato w/cheese	12.3 oz.	590	34.0	52

(continued)

FOOD	PORTION	TOTAL CALORIES	FAT (g)	CALORIES FROM FAT (%)
FAST FOODS—Continued				◆
Wendy's baked potato w/sour cream and chives	10.9 oz.	460	24.0	47
Wendy's french fries regular		300	15	45
FATS AND OILS				◆
Butter				
Regular, stick	1 Tbsp.	100	11.4	100 S
Whipped, tub	1 Tbsp.	65	7.3	100 S
Lard	1 Tbsp.	116	12.8	100 M,S
Margarine				
Diet corn	1 tsp.	17	1.9	100 P
Soft, corn or safflower	1 tsp.	34	3.8	100 P
Stick, regular or corn	1 tsp.	34	3.8	100 M
Whipped	1 tsp.	23	2.7	100 P
Oil				
Corn	1 Tbsp.	120	13.6	100 P
Olive	1 Tbsp.	119	13.5	100 M
Safflower	1 Tbsp.	120	13.6	100 P
Vegetable shortening	1 Tbsp.	113	12.8	100 M
FISH AND SEAFOOD				◆
Bluefish, baked w/butter	3 oz.	135	1.5	30
Clams				
Breaded, fried	3 oz.	183	9.9	49 M
Steamed	3 oz.	126	1.7	12
Cod, broiled w/butter	3.3 oz.	162	5.0	28
Crab				
Imperial	1 cup	323	16.7	47
Steamed	3 oz.	85	1.3	14

FOOD	PORTION	TOTAL CALORIES	FAT (g)	CALORIES FROM FAT (%)
Crab cake	1 (2 oz.)	93	4.5	44 M
Fish sticks, frozen	3 (1 oz.)	228	10.3	41 M
Flounder, baked	3 oz.	104	1.7	12
Haddock				
Baked	3 oz.	95	0.8	7
Breaded, fried	3 oz.	140	5.0	32
Halibut				
Broiled	3 oz.	119	2.5	19
Broiled w/butter	3 oz.	146	6.0	37
Lobster				
Broiled w/butter	1 tail (5 oz.)	134	10.8	73
Newburg	1 cup	485	26.5	49
Steamed	3 oz.	111	0.9	3
Thermidor	5.5 oz.	405	26.6	59
Mackerel				
Atlantic, canned	3 oz.	133	5.4	36 M
Broiled w/butter	3 oz.	197	13.4	62
Oysters				
Fried	3 oz.	167	10.7	58 M
On the half shell	3 oz.	117	4.2	32
Perch, breaded, fried	3 oz.	195	11.0	51 S
Red snapper, baked	3 oz.	104	1.7	12
Salmon				
Broiled w/butter	3.5 oz.	182	7.4	37
Canned	3 oz.	118	5.1	39 P
Salmon patty	3.5 oz.	239	12.4	47
Sardines				
In oil	1.3 oz.	75	4.1	50 P
In tomato sauce	1.3 oz.	68	4.6	60 M,P
Scallops				
Breaded, fried	3 oz.	183	9.9	49 M
Steamed	3 oz.	95	1.2	11

(continued)

THE FAT FIGHTER'S INDEX—Continued

FOOD	PORTION	TOTAL CALORIES	FAT (g)	CALORIES FROM FAT (%)

FISH AND SEAFOOD—Continued ♦

FOOD	PORTION	TOTAL CALORIES	FAT (g)	CALORIES FROM FAT (%)
Shrimp				
Breaded, fried	3 oz.	206	10.4	45
Steamed	3 oz.	84	0.9	10
Squid				
Fried	3 oz.	149	6.4	38 M
Raw	3 oz.	78	1.2	4
Surimi (imitation crab)	3 oz.	126	0.8	12
Swordfish, broiled w/butter	3.5 oz.	174	6.0	31
Trout, brook	3.5 oz.	196	11.2	51
Tuna, canned				
Diet	3 oz.	107	1.6	14
In oil	3 oz.	169	7.0	37 M,P
In water	3 oz.	111	0.4	3

FROZEN FOODS ♦

FOOD	PORTION	TOTAL CALORIES	FAT (g)	CALORIES FROM FAT (%)
Armour Classics Light				
Chicken Burgundy	10 oz.	190	2.0	9
Chicken Cacciatore w/rice and vegetables	11 oz.	250	4.0	14
Chicken Oriental	10.75 oz.	240	2.0	8
Salisbury Steak w/gravy, vegetables and potatoes	10.5 oz.	250	11.0	40
Sweet and Sour Chicken	10 oz.	180	1.0	5
Bird's Eye Pasta Side Dishes				
Italian Style Pasta	5 oz.	170	7.0	37
Noodles Stroganoff	5 oz.	180	9.0	45
Continental Style Pasta	5 oz.	160	9.0	51
Budget Gourmet Slim Selects Entrées				
Cheese Ravioli	10 oz.	290	10.0	31
Chicken Enchilada Suiza	8.75 oz.	290	12.0	37

FOOD	PORTION	TOTAL CALORIES	FAT (g)	CALORIES FROM FAT (%)
French Recipe Chicken and Vegetables	10 oz.	260	10.0	35
Lasagna w/meat sauce	10 oz.	290	10.0	31
Sirloin of Beef in herb sauce	9.5 oz.	220	7.0	29
Sirloin Salisbury Steak	8.5 oz.	280	15.0	48
Green Giant Pasta Accents				
Creamy Cheddar	½ cup	100	5.0	45
Garden Herb	½ cup	80	3.0	33
Pasta Primavera	½ cup	110	5.0	41
Health Valley Lean Living				
Cheese Enchiladas	9 oz.	280	5.0	16
Chicken à la King	9 oz.	380	17.0	40
Chicken Crepes	9 oz.	380	22.0	52
Spinach Lasagna	9 oz.	170	3.0	16
Lean Cuisine				
Beef and Pork Canneloni w/Mornay Sauce	9.62 oz.	270	10.0	33
Breast of Chicken Marsala w/vegetables	8.12 oz.	190	5.0	24
Cheese Cannelloni w/tomato sauce	9.62 oz.	270	10.0	33
Chicken à l'Orange w/Almond Rice	8 oz.	270	5.0	17
Chicken and Vegetables w/vermicelli	12.75 oz.	270	7.0	23
Chicken Chow Mein w/rice	11.25 oz.	250	5.0	18
Filet of Fish Jardiniere w/souffléed potatoes	11.25 oz.	280	10.0	32
Linguini w/clam sauce	9.62 oz.	260	7.0	24
Oriental Scallops w/vegetables and rice	8.62 oz.	220	3.0	12

(continued)

253

THE FAT FIGHTER'S INDEX—Continued

FOOD	PORTION	TOTAL CALORIES	FAT (g)	CALORIES FROM FAT (%)
FROZEN FOODS—Continued				◆
Lean Pockets				
Chicken Parmesan	5 oz.	270	6.0	20
Pizza Deluxe	5 oz.	280	13.0	41
Le Menu Light Style				
Beef à l'Orange	10 oz.	290	8.0	25
Chicken Cacciatore	10 oz.	260	8.0	28
Country Mustard Pasta Salad				
w/Swiss Cheese	8 oz.	270	10.0	33
Creamy Dill Pasta Salad				
w/tuna	8 oz.	260	8.0	28
Creamy Tarragon Pasta Salad				
w/chicken	7.75 oz.	240	7.0	26
Flounder Vin Blanc	10 oz.	220	5.0	20
Glazed Chicken Breast	10 oz.	240	5.0	19
Oriental Pasta Salad w/chicken	8.75 oz.	240	4.0	15
Salisbury Steak w/Italian-style				
sauce and vegetables	9.5 oz.	270	13.0	43
Salsa Mexicana Pasta Salad				
w/turkey	8.37 oz.	260	6.0	21
Spaghetti w/beef				
and mushroom sauce	11.5 oz.	280	7.0	23
3-Cheese Stuffed Shells	10 oz.	280	8.0	26
Turkey Dijon	9.5 oz.	280	10.0	32
Turkey Divan	10 oz.	280	9.0	29
Zesty Italian Pasta Salad				
w/cheese and salami	7.63 oz	270	8.0	27
Zucchini Lasagna	11 oz.	260	7.0	24
Microwave Garden Gourmet				
Fettucine Primavera	9.5 oz.	230	8.0	31
Pasta Florentine	9.5 oz.	230	9.0	35
Rotini Cheddar	9.5 oz.	230	10.0	39
Tortellini Provencale	9.5 oz.	210	5.0	21

FOOD	PORTION	TOTAL CALORIES	FAT (g)	CALORIES FROM FAT (%)
Minute Microwave (as packaged w/out optional butter added)				
Chicken Flavored Noodles	½ cup	150	2.0	12
Noodles Alfredo	½ cup	150	3.0	18
Parmesan Noodles	½ cup	140	3.0	19
Mrs. Paul's Light				
Seafood Entrées				
Fish au Gratin	10 oz.	290	8.0	25
Fish Dijon	9.5 oz.	280	15.0	48
Fish Florentine	9 oz.	210	4.0	17
Fish Mornay	10 oz.	280	14.0	45
Fish and Pasta				
Florentine	9.5 oz.	240	9.0	34
Shrimp and Clams w/linguini	10 oz.	280	6.0	19
Shrimp Cajun Style	10.5 oz.	200	4.0	18
Shrimp Oriental	11 oz.	280	5.0	16
Shrimp Primavera	11 oz.	240	4.0	15
Tuna Pasta Casserole	11 oz.	290	7.0	22
Weight Watchers				
Beef Salisbury Steak				
Romana w/noodles	8.75 oz.	320	11.0	31
Cheese Enchiladas Ranchero	8.87 oz.	370	23.0	56
Cheese French Bread Pizza	5.12 oz.	320	13.0	37
Chicken à la King	9 oz.	220	7.0	29
Chicken Cacciatore				
w/spaghetti	10.5 oz.	300	6.0	18
Chicken Nuggets	4 (3 oz.)	180	10.0	50
Chicken Patty Parmigiana				
w/vegetables	8.06 oz.	280	15.0	48
Deluxe Combination Pizza	6.75 oz.	280	6.0	19
Fillet of Fish				
au Gratin w/broccoli	9.25 oz.	220	6.0	25
Imperial Chicken w/rice	9.25 oz.	220	5.0	20

(continued)

THE FAT FIGHTER'S INDEX—Continued

FOOD	PORTION	TOTAL CALORIES	FAT (g)	CALORIES FROM FAT (%)
FROZEN FOODS—Continued				◆
Oven-Fried Fish	6.81 oz.	220	12.0	49
Pasta Rigati	11 oz.	290	8.0	25
Seafood Linguini w/noodles	9 oz.	220	7.0	29
Southern Fried Chicken				
Patty w/vegetables	6.5 oz.	270	16.0	53
Sweet 'n Sour				
Chicken Tenders w/rice	10.19 oz.	250	2.0	7
Stuffed Sole w/Newburg Sauce	10.5 oz.	270	8.0	27
Stuffed Turkey Breast				
w/vegetables	8.5 oz.	260	10.0	35
FRUITS AND JUICES				◆
Apple	5 oz.	81	0.5	5
Apricot, raw	1 (1.25 oz.)	17	0.1	7
Avocado				
California	1 (6 oz.)	306	30.0	88 M
Florida	1 (6 oz.)	193	15.4	72 M
Banana	1 (4 oz.)	105	0.6	5
Berries				
Blackberries	1 cup	74	0.6	7
Blueberries	1 cup	82	0.6	6
Raspberries	1 cup	61	0.7	10
Strawberries	1 cup	45	0.6	11
Cherries				
Sour	1 cup	72	0.7	9
Sweet	1 cup	105	1.5	12
Cranberry sauce	¼ cup	105	0.1	1

FOOD	PORTION	TOTAL CALORIES	FAT (g)	CALORIES FROM FAT (%)
Dried fruit				
Apples	1 cup	209	0.3	1
Figs	1 cup	508	2.3	4
Prunes	1 cup	385	0.8	2
Raisins	1 cup	434	0.7	1
Figs	1 (.75 oz.)	37	0.2	4
Fruit cocktail	¼ cup	47	0.1	1
Grapefruit	1 (8 oz.)	72	0.2	3
Grapes	1 cup	58	0.3	5
Juice				
Apple	1 cup	116	0.3	2
Cranberry	1 cup	147	0.1	1
Cranapple	1 cup	180	0.1	1
Grape	1 cup	155	0.2	1
Grapefruit	1 cup	96	0.3	2
Orange	1 cup	111	0.5	4
Pineapple	1 cup	139	0.2	1
Prune	1 cup	181	0.1	1
Kiwifruit	1	46	0.3	7
Lemon	1 (2 oz.)	17	0.2	9
Mango	1 (7 oz.)	135	0.6	4
Melon				
Casaba	1 cup	45	0.2	3
Cantaloupe	1 cup	57	0.4	7
Watermelon	1 cup	50	0.7	12
Nectarine	1 (5 oz.)	67	0.6	8
Orange, all varieties	1 (4.5 oz.)	62	0.2	2
Papaya	1 cup	54	0.2	3
Peach	1	37	0.1	2
Pear, Bartlett	1 (6 oz.)	98	0.7	6
Pineapple, diced	1 cup	77	0.7	8
Plum, Japanese	1	36	0.4	10

(continued)

THE FAT FIGHTER'S INDEX—Continued

FOOD	PORTION	TOTAL CALORIES	FAT (g)	CALORIES FROM FAT (%)
GRAIN PRODUCTS				◆
Bulgur, dry	½ cup	314	1.3	4
Noodles				
Chow mein	1 cup	220	11.0	45
Egg	1 cup	200	2.0	9
Ramen	1 cup	207	8.6	37
Oyster crackers	5	9	0.3	25
Pearl barley, dry	½ cup	350	1.0	3
Rice				
Brown	½ cup	110	0.9	7
Brown, basmati	½ cup	85	0.1	1
White	½ cup	103	0	0
White, basmati	½ cup	82	0	0
Wild	⅓ cup	50	0	0
Saltines	5	63	1.3	18
Spaghetti or macaroni	1 cup	173	1.0	5
Stuffing, prepared mix	½ cup	70	3.0	39
Taco shell	1	50	2.2	39
Tortilla, corn or flour	1	81	1.5	16
MEATS				◆
Beef				
Chicken-fried steak	3.5 oz.	389	30.0	69
Chipped, dried	2.5 oz.	117	2.8	21
Corned beef, canned	3 oz.	213	12.7	54 M,S
Corned beef hash	¼ cup	100	6.3	56 S
Eye round roast	3 oz.	155	5.5	32 M,S
Ground, 10% fat	3 oz.	217	13.9	58 M,S
Ground, 21% fat	3 oz.	231	15.7	61 M,S
Ground, up to 30% fat, baked or broiled	3 oz.	244	17.8	66 M,S

FOOD	PORTION	TOTAL CALORIES	FAT (g)	CALORIES FROM FAT (%)
Ground, up to 30% fat, fried	3 oz.	260	19.2	66 M,S
Liver, fried	3 oz.	184	6.8	33 S
London broil, top round	3 oz.	162	5.3	29 M,S
Pot roast	3.5 oz.	231	10.0	39 M,S
Rib roast, trimmed	3 oz.	203	11.7	52 M,S
Rib steak	3.5 oz.	225	11.6	46 M,S
Roast beef, lean, trimmed	3 oz.	189	8.7	41 M,S
Sirloin steak, trimmed, broiled	3 oz.	202	10.1	45 M,S
Tenderloin, broiled	3 oz.	174	7.9	41 M,S
Frankfurters				
Beef or pork	1	183	16.6	82 M,S
Beef or pork w/cheese	1	141	12.5	80 M,S
Frog legs, fried	1 oz.	82	5.6	62
Lamb				
Chop, broiled	3 oz.	360	32.0	80 S
Leg, roasted, trimmed	3 oz.	156	6.0	35 S
Shoulder, lean	3 oz.	173	8.0	42 S
Pork				
Chitterlings	1 oz.	86	8.2	85 M,S
Ham, canned, roasted	3 oz.	193	12.9	60 M,S
Ham, extra lean	3 oz.	116	4.1	32 M,S
Ham, roasted, w/bone	3 oz.	151	7.7	46 M,S
Chop, trimmed	3 oz.	218	13.0	54 M,S
Loin, trimmed, roasted	3 oz.	213	11.6	49 M,S
Shoulder, lean, roasted	3 oz.	207	12.8	55 M,S
Spareribs, braised	3 oz.	338	25.7	68 M,S
Tenderloin, roasted	3 oz.	141	4.1	26 M,S
Rabbit, stewed	3 oz.	183	8.6	42
Sausage				
Bratwurst	3 oz	256	22.0	77 M,S

(continued)

THE FAT FIGHTER'S INDEX—Continued

FOOD	PORTION	TOTAL CALORIES	FAT (g)	CALORIES FROM FAT (%)
MEATS—Continued				◆
Sausages—continued				
Italian, pork	3 oz.	275	21.8	71 M,S
Kielbasa	3 oz.	265	23.1	78 M,S
Knockwurst, pork/beef	1 (2.4 oz.)	209	18.9	81 M,S
Polish, pork	3 oz.	277	24.4	79 M,S
Vienna, canned, pork/beef	1 link	45	4.0	81 M,S
Veal				
Cutlet, broiled	3 oz.	185	9.0	44 M,S
Rib, roasted	3 oz.	230	14.0	55 S
Venison, roasted	3.5 oz.	146	2.2	14
NUTS AND SEEDS				◆
Almonds, dry roasted, whole	1 cup	810	71.3	79 M
Brazil nuts	1 cup	919	92.7	91 M,P
Cashews, dry roasted	1 cup	787	63.5	73 M
Chestnuts, roasted	1 oz.	68	0.3	5 M
Coconut				
Dry, flaked	1 cup	341	24.4	64 S
Raw, shredded	1 cup	283	26.8	85
Filberts (hazelnuts)	1 cup	727	72.0	89 M
Macadamia nuts	1 cup	940	98.8	95 M
Peanuts, dry roasted w/out salt	1 cup	867	76.5	79 M
Pecans	1 cup	721	73.1	91 M,P
Pistachios, dry roasted	1 cup	776	67.6	78 M
Sesame seeds, dried	1 cup	825	71.5	78 P
Sunflower seeds				
Dried	1 cup	821	71.4	78 P
Oil-roasted	1 cup	830	77.6	84 P
Walnuts, English	1 cup	770	74.2	87 P

FOOD	PORTION	TOTAL CALORIES	FAT (g)	CALORIES FROM FAT (%)
POULTRY				♦
Chicken				
Capon, roasted	3 oz.	194	9.9	46 M
Breast, batter-fried	½	364	18.5	46 M
Breast, roasted	½	193	7.7	36 M
Breast, roasted w/out skin	½	142	3.0	19 M,S
Leg, roasted	1 (4 oz.)	265	15.4	52 M
Leg, roasted w/out skin	1 (4 oz.)	218	9.6	40 M
Liver, simmered	3 oz.	133	4.6	31 S
Liver paté	1 Tbsp.	26	1.7	59
Duck				
Roasted	3 oz.	286	24.1	76 M,S
Roasted w/out skin	3 oz.	171	9.5	50 M,S
Turkey				
Breast, roasted w/out skin	3 oz.	115	0.6	5 S,P
Leg, roasted w/out skin	3 oz.	135	3.2	21 S,P
Turkey or chicken roll, light or dark	1 oz.	43	2.1	43 M
SAUCES, GRAVIES, AND DRESSINGS				♦
Dressings				
Blue cheese, Italian, or Russian	1 Tbsp.	74	7.6	90 P
Blue cheese, low-calorie	1 Tbsp.	10	1.0	93 S
French, low-calorie	1 Tbsp.	22	0.9	37 P
French or thousand island	1 Tbsp.	63	6.0	86 P
Italian, low-calorie	1 Tbsp.	16	1.5	85 P
Ranch-style	1 Tbsp.	54	5.7	95
Sweet-and-sour	1 Tbsp.	29	0.3	9
Vinegar and oil	1 Tbsp.	72	8.0	100 P

(continued)

THE FAT FIGHTER'S INDEX—Continued

FOOD	PORTION	TOTAL CALORIES	FAT (g)	CALORIES FROM FAT (%)
SAUCES, GRAVIES, AND DRESSINGS—Continued				◆
Gravies				
Beef, canned	1 Tbsp.	8	0.3	40 S
Chicken, canned	1 Tbsp.	12	0.9	65 M
Mushroom	1 Tbsp.	8	0.4	48 M,P
Pork, mix	1 Tbsp.	5	0.1	23 M,S
Turkey, canned	1 Tbsp.	8	0.3	37 M
Sauces				
Barbecue	1 Tbsp.	12	0.3	22 M,P
Béarnaise or hollandaise, mix	1 Tbsp.	44	4.3	87 S
Cheese, mix, w/milk	1 Tbsp.	19	1.1	50 S
Chili	1 Tbsp.	16	0	0
Curry, mix	1 Tbsp.	17	0.9	49 S
Marinara, canned	¼ cup	43	2.1	44 M
Sour cream, mix	1 Tbsp.	32	1.9	54 S
Spaghetti, canned	¼ cup	68	3.0	39 M
Stroganoff, mix	1 Tbsp.	17	0.7	36 S
Taco, canned	¼ cup	22	1.4	57
Tartar	1 Tbsp.	75	8.0	96 S
Tomato, canned	¼ cup	19	0.1	5 M,S
White	1 Tbsp.	25	1.9	69 S
SNACKS				◆
Corn chips	1 oz.	155	9.1	53 P,M
Crackers				
Animal	1	9	0.2	21
Cheese	1	5	0.3	55 S
Graham, plain	1	28	0.5	16 M
Rye	1	9	0.4	37
Wheat	1	9	0.4	35
Hummus	1 Tbsp.	26	1.3	45
Peanuts, honey roasted	1 oz.	170	12.0	64

262

FOOD	PORTION	TOTAL CALORIES	FAT (g)	CALORIES FROM FAT (%)
Popcorn				
Homemade, plain	1 cup	25	0	0
Microwave, plain	1⅓ cups	110	7.0	57
W/oil and salt	1 cup	40	2.0	45
Potato chip	1	11	0.7	61 P
Pretzels	1	60	1.0	15
Rice cake	1	35	0.3	7
Tortilla chips	1 oz.	139	6.6	43 M

SOUPS ◆

FOOD	PORTION	TOTAL CALORIES	FAT (g)	CALORIES FROM FAT (%)
Bean w/bacon, canned	1 cup	173	5.9	31
Beef noodle, canned	1 cup	84	3.1	33
Beef stock				
Canned	1 cup	16	0.5	30 S
Homemade	average	333	21.0	57 M,S
Cauliflower, homemade	1 cup	196	8.7	40
Celery, canned, w/milk	1 cup	165	9.7	53
Chicken noodle, homemade	1 cup	184	2.7	13
Chicken stock				
Canned	1 cup	39	1.4	32 M
Homemade	1 cup	166	10.3	56 M,S
Clam chowder				
Manhattan	1 cup	78	2.3	27 M,P
New England	1 cup	163	6.6	36
Cream of chicken, canned	1 cup	191	11.5	54 M
Cream of mushroom	1 cup	203	13.6	60 P
Cream of mushroom, diet	10.5 oz.	90	2.0	20 S,P
Gazpacho				
Canned	1 cup	57	2.2	35 P
Homemade	1 cup	116	7.1	55 P
Minestrone	1 cup	83	2.5	27
Onion, canned	1 cup	57	1.7	27

(continued)

263

THE FAT FIGHTER'S INDEX—Continued

FOOD	PORTION	TOTAL CALORIES	FAT (g)	CALORIES FROM FAT (%)
SOUPS—Continued				◆
Oyster stew, canned, w/milk	1 cup	134	7.9	53 S
Pea, green				
Canned	1 cup	239	7.0	66 S
Homemade	1 cup	296	7.0	21
Tomato, canned				
W/milk	1 cup	160	6.0	34 S
W/water	1 cup	86	1.9	20 P
Vegetable, canned	1 cup	72	1.9	24 M,P
Vegetable w/barley	1 cup	99	4.4	40 P,M
Vegetable beef, canned	1 cup	79	1.9	22 S,M
Vegetable stock, homemade	1 cup	83	0.4	4
VEGETABLES				◆
Alfalfa sprouts	1 cup	10	0.2	21 P
Artichoke, boiled	4.2 oz.	53	0.2	3 P
Asparagus				
Boiled	1 cup	44	0.6	11 P
Canned	1 cup	48	1.6	29 P
Beans				
Garbanzo, canned	1 oz.	28	0.5	17
Green or wax, boiled	1 cup	44	0.4	7 P
Lima, boiled	1 cup	208	0.5	2 P
Beets, canned	1 cup	54	0.2	4 P
Broccoli				
Boiled	1 cup	46	0.4	9 P
Raw	1 cup	24	0.3	11 P
Brussels sprouts, boiled	1 cup	60	0.8	12 P
Cabbage				
Boiled	1 cup	31	0.4	11 P
Red, raw	1 cup	19	0.2	9 P

FOOD	PORTION	TOTAL CALORIES	FAT (g)	CALORIES FROM FAT (%)
Carrot, raw	1 (2.5 oz.)	31	0.1	4 P
Cauliflower, raw	1 cup	24	0.2	7
Celery	1 stalk	6	0.1	8 P
Chard, boiled	1 cup	35	0.1	4
Corn				
Canned	1 cup	132	1.6	11 P
Fresh, boiled	1 ear (2.7 oz.)	83	1.0	11 P
Lettuce				
Iceberg	4.8 oz.	18	0.3	13 P
Romaine	1 cup	8	0.1	14 P
Mushrooms, raw	1 cup	18	0.3	15 P
Onions				
Chopped	1 cup	54	0.4	7 P
Ring, fried	1	41	3.0	59 M,S
Peas				
Boiled	1 cup	126	0.4	3 P
Split, dried, cooked	1 cup	230	1.0	4
Pepper, sweet	1 (2.6 oz.)	18	0.3	17 P
Potatoes				
Baked	1 (7 oz.)	220	0.2	1 P,S
French fried	3 oz.	187	7.5	36 S,M
Hash brown	½ cup	170	9.0	47 M,S
Mashed w/milk and butter	1 cup	222	8.9	36 M
Sweet, baked	4 oz.	118	0.1	1 P
Sweet, candied	1 (3.7 oz.)	144	3.4	21 S
Radishes	6	4	0.1	31 P
Sauerkraut, canned	1 cup	44	0.3	7 P
Spinach				
Canned	1 cup	50	1.1	19 P
Creamed, frozen	4.5 oz.	190	15.0	71
Raw	1 cup	12	0.2	15 P
Squash, acorn, baked	1 cup	115	0.3	2 P

(continued)

THE FAT FIGHTER'S INDEX—Continued

FOOD	PORTION	TOTAL CALORIES	FAT (g)	CALORIES FROM FAT (%)
VEGETABLES—Continued				◆
Tomatoes				
Canned	1 cup	47	0.6	11 P
Stewed, homemade	1 cup	59	2.2	34 M
Watercress	1 cup	4	0.1	9 P,S
Zucchini, boiled	1 cup	28	0.1	3 P

SOURCES: *Food Values: Cholesterol and Fats* by Leah Wallach, U.S. Department of Agriculture, National Research Council, manufacturers' data.

INDEX

Page references in *italic* indicate tables.